Critical Reviews in
Toxicology

Volume 26 / Issue 2   1996

Special Issue

Tobacco-Specific N-Nitrosamines: Recent Advances

This book is a reproduction of Critical Reviews in Toxicology, Volume 26, Issue 2. Due to the sequencing of articles for the volume, the pages have been numbered to reflect this.

Anita Klein: Senior Typesetter

CRC Press
Taylor & Francis Group
6000 Broken Sound Parkway NW, Suite 300
Boca Raton, FL 33487-2742

© 1996 by Taylor & Francis Group, LLC
CRC Press is an imprint of Taylor & Francis Group, an Informa business

First issued in paperback 2019

No claim to original U.S. Government works

ISBN 13: 978-0-367-44857-8 (pbk)
ISBN 13: 978-0-8493-1156-7 (hbk)

Visit the Taylor & Francis Web site at
http://www.taylorandfrancis.com

and the CRC Press Web site at
http://www.crcpress.com

Critical Reviews in Toxicology is covered in *Current Contents/Life Sciences,* the Scisearch® online database, the *Research Alert* service, and the *Science Citation Index;* abstracted and indexed in the BIOSIS Database and in *Current Awareness in Biological Sciences;* abstracted in *Cambridge Scientific Abstracts* and in *Chemical Abstracts Service;* and indexed in *Environmental Periodicals Bibliography.*

Critical Reviews in
Toxicology

Volume 26 / Issue 2 1996

CRITICAL REVIEWS IN TOXICOLOGY

AIMS & SCOPE

Provides up-to-date, objective analyses of important topics, based on the work of a triumvirate: the author, an acknowledged authority in the field; the referee, capable of undertaking a critical appraisal of the strengths and weaknesses of the review; and the editor who attempts to ensure that the crucial issues of special importance are given adequate attention.

Activity is aimed at making available critical assessments of subjects that are part of the advancing frontiers of toxicology and related basic scientific disciplines; or issues that form the core of some of the most complex and intractable problems with which the toxicologist has to grapple.

Tobacco-Specific *N*-Nitrosamines: Recent Advances

TABLE OF CONTENTS

INTRODUCTION

The proceedings of the 15th International Cancer Congress held in August 1990 in Hamburg, Germany, included a round table discussion on "Tobacco-Specific *N*-Nitrosamines (TSNA)".[1] Four years later, the Program Committee for the 16th International Cancer Congress, held in October-November 1994 in New Delhi, India, deemed it of importance and of general interest to have a symposium on TSNA. As Hecht pointed out, there have been during the 5 years preceding the Symposium more than 100 scientific publications on the chemistry, biochemistry, bioassays, and molecular biology of the highly carcinogenic 4-(methylnitrosamino)-1-(3-pyridyl)-1-butanone (NNK) alone. As this reflects the significance of the TSNA to the cancer research community,[2] the participants of this symposium greatly appreciate the decision of the editors of *Critical Reviews in Toxicology* to assign a special issue of the journal to the papers presented at the TSNA Symposium.

In 1962, Druckrey had suggested that nicotine as a precursor for *N*-nitrosamines may play an important role in tobacco carcinogenesis.[3] Twenty-eight years later, in 1994, when Herman Druckrey passed away, his ideas and concept have been richly confirmed. Nicotine is not only the major pharmacoactive agent in tobacco, but it gives rise to several TSNA during tobacco processing and smoking, and these TSNA include the highly carcinogenic NNK and *N*′-nitrosonornicotine (NNN). The six presentations on TSNA published in this issue of *Critical Reviews in Toxicology* will inform the readers about the current state of knowledge and the progress achieved. This summary points to the research tasks that remain to be carried out before we can fully evaluate the contribution of TSNA to human cancer.

Dietrich Hoffmann
American Health Foundation
Valhalla, NY

REFERENCES

1. **Hoffmann, D. and Spiegelhalder, B.,** Tobacco-specific *N*-nitrosamines, *Crit. Rev. Toxicol.,* 21(4), 1991.

2. **Hecht, S. S.,** Recent studies on mechanisms of bioactivation and detoxification of 4-(methylnitrosamino)-1-(3-pyridyl)-1-butanone, *Crit. Rev. Toxicol.,* 1996 (this issue).

3. **Druckrey, H. and Preussmann, R.,** Zur Entstehung carcinogener Nitrosamine am Beispiel des Tabakrauches, *Naturwissenschaften,* 49, 498, 1962.

FORMATION AND ANALYSIS OF TOBACCO-SPECIFIC *N*-NITROSAMINES

Critical Reviews in Toxicology, 26(2):121–137 (1996)

Formation and Analysis of Tobacco-Specific N-Nitrosamines

Klaus D. Brunnemann, Bogdan Prokopczyk, Mirjana V. Djordjevic, and Dietrich Hoffmann

Naylor Dana Institute for Disease Prevention, American Health Foundation, Valhalla, NY 10595.

ABSTRACT: Chemical-analytical studies during the past 4 years led to several new observations on the formation of tobacco-specific N-nitrosamines (TSNA) and their occurrence in smokeless tobacco, mainstream smoke (MS), and sidestream smoke (SS) of American and foreign cigarettes. When snuff was extracted by means of supercritical fluid extraction with carbon dioxide containing 10% methanol, analysis of this material confirmed that the extraction with organic solvents had been partially incomplete.

Epidemiological studies in the northern Sudan showed a high risk for oral cancer for users of toombak, a home-made oral snuff. Toombak contains 100-fold higher levels of TSNA than commercial snuff in the U.S. and Sweden. The TSNA content in the saliva of toombak dippers is at least ten times higher than that reported in the saliva of dippers of commercial snuff. Biomarker studies have shown corresponding high levels of hemoglobin adducts with metabolites of NNN and NNK as well as for urinary metabolites of NNK. These data supported the epidemiological findings.

The analyses of MS of U.S. and foreign cigarettes smoked under FTC conditions revealed comparable data for the smoke of nonfilter cigarettes and filter cigarettes except in the case of low- and ultralow-yield cigarettes, which showed reduced TSNA yields. The MS of cigarettes made from Burley or dark tobacco is exceptionally high in TSNA, primarily because of the high nitrate content of those tobacco types. Taking puffs of larger volume and drawing puffs more frequently, practices observed among most smokers of cigarettes with low nicotine yield, results in high TSNA values in the MS. The formation of the lung carcinogen NNK is favored during the smoldering of cigarettes, between puffs, when SS is generated. Consequently, in most samples from indoor air polluted with environmental tobacco smoke (ETS), the highest concentration of an individual TSNA is that of NNK. When nonsmokers had remained for up to 2 h in a test laboratory with high ETS pollution, they excreted measurable amounts of NNK metabolites in the urine, indicative of the uptake of TSNA.

KEY WORDS: gas chromatography (GC), thermal energy analyzer (TEA), supercritical fluid extraction (SFE), snuff, cigarette mainstream smoke (MS), sidestream smoke (SS), tobacco-specific N-nitrosamines (TSNA), N'-nitrosonornicotine (NNN), 4-(methyl-nitrosamino)-1-(3-pyridyl)-1-butanone (NNK).

I. INTRODUCTION

During the past few years, biochemical, molecular-biological, and biomarker studies have greatly enhanced the concept that the tobacco-specific N-nitrosamines (TSNA) are major contributors to the increased risk of snuff dippers for cancer of the upper digestive tract and the risk of smokers for cancer of the respiratory tract and pancreas.[1] These aspects are discussed in the subsequent presentations of this symposium.

1040-8444/96/$.50

Since the International Cancer Congress in Hamburg, Germany, in 1990, new knowledge has been gathered as to the formation of TSNA (Figure 1) and new methods for the analysis of these carcinogens in tobacco and tobacco smoke have been developed. In this presentation, we describe these new insights and developments.

II. FORMATION OF TSNA

Figure 2 presents the formation of TSNA by nitrosation of secondary and tertiary amines. Tobacco alkaloids with a secondary amino group are nornicotine, anatabine, anabasine, and (likely also) cotinine acid; among those with a tertiary amino group is the major tobacco alkaloid nicotine (Figure 1). An earlier study had shown that at ambient temperature and at a range between pH 2 and 7, nicotine is nitrosated to N'-nitrosonornicotine (NNN), 4-(methylnitrosamino)-4-(3-pyridyl)-butanal (NNA) and 4-(methylnitrosamino)-1-(3-pyridyl)-1-butanone (NNK).[2] The rate of nicotine nitrosation is slow, as it is for tertiary amines in general.[3,4] The rate-limiting step is the formation of the iminium intermediate (Figure 2). Adding thiocyanate, a catalyst present in physiological fluids especially of smokers, doubles the rate of N-nitrosation of nicotine.[3] The nitrosation kinetics of the minor tobacco alkaloids nornicotine and anabasine follows those of aliphatic secondary amines. Despite the different rate constants for the N-nitrosation of nicotine and nornicotine, most NNN in tobacco stems from nicotine rather than from nornicotine.[5]

The TSNA in smokeless tobacco are primarily formed after harvesting of the leaves during drying, curing, aging, and es-

Formation of Tobacco-Specific Nitrosamines

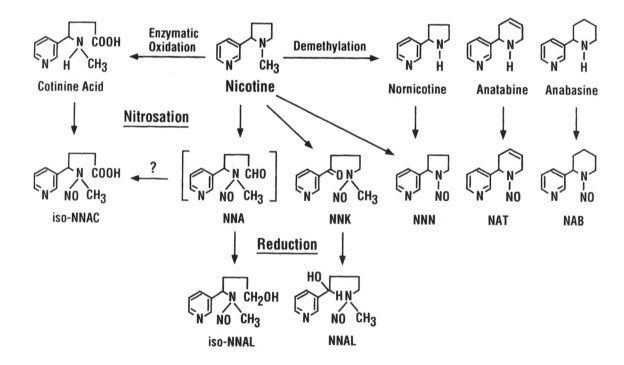

FIGURE 1. Formation of tobacco-specific nitrosamines.

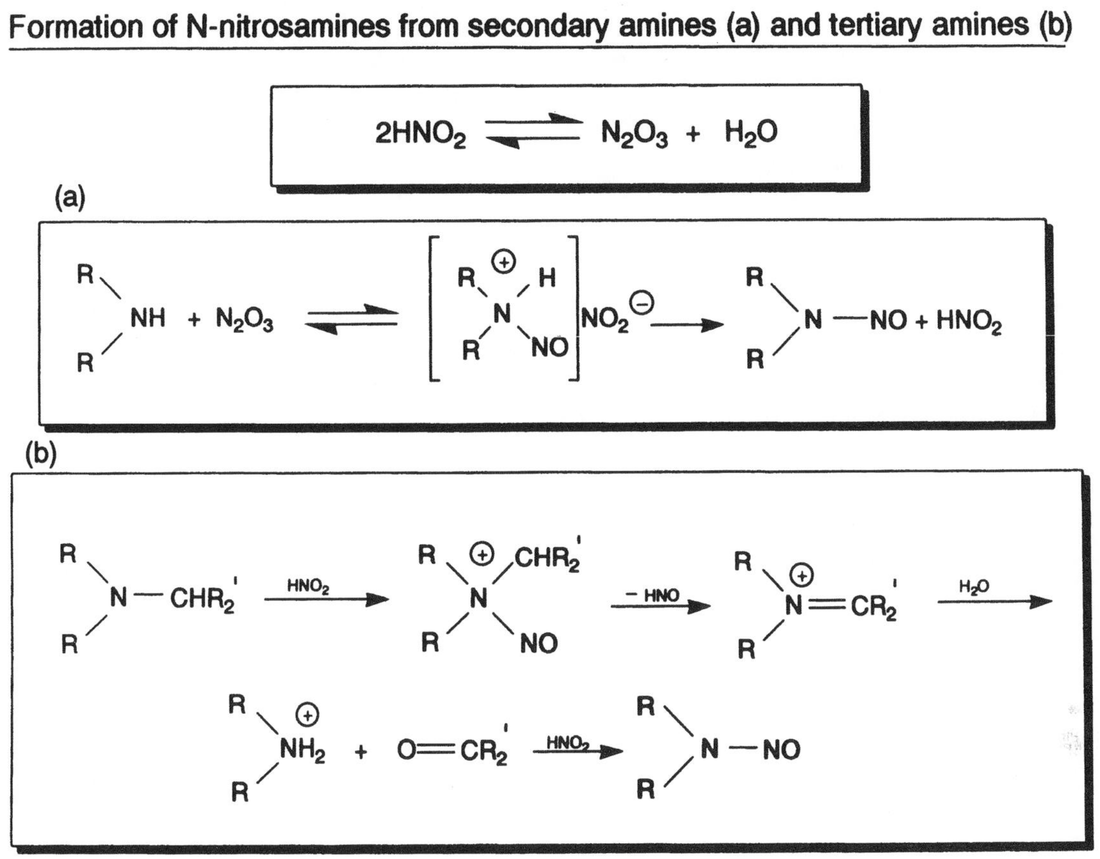

Formation of N-nitrosamines from secondary amines (a) and tertiary amines (b)

$$2HNO_2 \rightleftharpoons N_2O_3 + H_2O$$

(a)

$$\begin{array}{c} R \\ \diagdown \\ NH \\ \diagup \\ R \end{array} + N_2O_3 \rightleftharpoons \left[\begin{array}{c} R \quad \overset{\oplus}{} \quad H \\ \diagdown N \diagup \\ \diagup \quad \diagdown \\ R \quad NO \end{array} \right] NO_2^{\ominus} \longrightarrow \begin{array}{c} R \\ \diagdown \\ N-NO + HNO_2 \\ \diagup \\ R \end{array}$$

(b)

$$\begin{array}{c} R \\ \diagdown \\ N-CHR_2' \\ \diagup \\ R \end{array} \xrightarrow{HNO_2} \begin{array}{c} R \quad \overset{\oplus}{} \quad CHR_2' \\ \diagdown N \diagup \\ \diagup \quad \diagdown \\ R \quad NO \end{array} \xrightarrow{-HNO} \begin{array}{c} R \quad \overset{\oplus}{} \\ \diagdown N=CR_2' \\ \diagup \\ R \end{array} \xrightarrow{H_2O}$$

$$\begin{array}{c} R \\ \diagdown \overset{\oplus}{} \\ NH_2 \\ \diagup \\ R \end{array} + O=CR_2' \xrightarrow{HNO_2} \begin{array}{c} R \\ \diagdown \\ N-NO \\ \diagup \\ R \end{array}$$

FIGURE 2. Formation of N-nitrosamines from secondary amines (a) and tertiary amines (b).

pecially during fermentation. Model studies with reference snuff and with commercial snuff brands have clearly documented that during storage at ambient and at elevated temperatures for longer than 4 weeks, additional amounts of TNSA are formed.[6-10] This additional formation of TSNA during the storage of smokeless tobacco may be a major factor for the broad ranges of nitrite nitrogen (RSD: 27 to 65%), NNN (RSD: 10 to 20%), and NNK (RSD: 10 to 33%) content of the five leading U.S. brands bought in different areas of the U.S. Furthermore, the yields of nitrite and TSNA vary greatly among the five best-selling brands. The leading snuff brand (42% of 1993 sales) contains 672 ± 297 ppm nitrite nitrogen, 8.73 ± 1.44 ppm NNN, and 1.89 ± 0.62 ppm NNK, while the fourth-best-selling snuff brand (2% of

the 1993 market) has 1.3 ± 0.4 ppm nitrite nitrogen, 5.09 ± 1.03 ppm NNN, and 0.92 ± 0.26 ppm of NNK. The yields of TSNA in the five leading U.S. snuff brands are highly significantly correlated with the nitrite content ($p = 0.003$) but not with the nitrate content ($p > 0.05$).[11]

During the last decade, the levels of TSNA determined in analyses of the major U.S. snuff brands have shown a remarkable decrease by 70 to 92%; in the Swedish leading snuff brands, this trend has occurred for the last 2 decades.[12] Such reduction has been primarily achieved by changing the processing of tobacco into snuff, most notably by modifying the fermentation step. Recent model studies have also shown that treating tobacco leaves directly after harvesting with strains of certain bacteria that reduce nitrate and/or nitrite to ammonia will significantly inhibit TSNA formation during tobacco processing.[13]

III. ANALYSIS OF TSNA

A few years ago we made the observation that even after repeated organic solvent extractions of TSNA from snuff, the residual tobacco released additional amounts of NNK when incubated with saliva.[14] This suggested that NNK, but not NNN, NAB, or NAT, is in some way more strongly bound to the tobacco leaf and is not readily released after extraction with organic solvents; thus, the conventional analytical method using organic solvents for the extraction appeared to be incomplete. This was confirmed when we employed supercritical fluid extraction (SFE) for the determination of TSNA in tobacco.[15,16] In SFE, freeze-dried tobacco that contains 4.0 to 4.5% water is placed in an extraction vessel with ethyl-NNK as an internal standard. The vessel is then heated to 60°C and pressurized to 350 atm with carbon dioxide that contains 10% methanol. The extracted analyte is collected in n-hexane. The residue is cleaned up on a small silica gel cartridge, and the eluate is analyzed by gas chromatography with a thermal energy analyzer (GC-TEA) using N-nitrosoguvacoline (NG) as a chromatographic standard (Figure 3). The recovery of the TSNA is greater than 90% and is well reproducible. Table 1 compares the analytical data for TSNA in three moist snuff samples obtained with the conventional solvent extraction and with SFE.[16]

IV. TOOMBAK, A HOME-MADE SNUFF IN THE NORTHERN SUDAN

Surveys of the population of the northern provinces of the Sudan have shown high incidence rates of cancer of the upper diges-

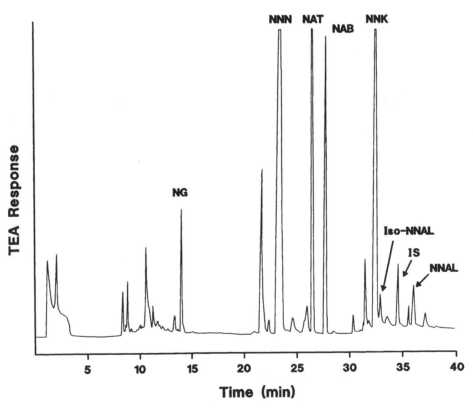

FIGURE 3. Representative GC-TEA chromatogram of *N*-Nitrosamines from Sudanese snuff (Toombak).

TABLE 1
Comparison of the Conventional Solvent Extraction Method with a New Improved Methodology Utilizing Supercritical Solvent Extraction[a]

| Toombak | Levels of TSNA in toombak (μg/g dry weight)[b] | | | | | |
	NNN	NAT	NAB	NNK	*iso*-NNAL	NNAL
A						
SFE	141	21.7	28.7	245	10.9	22.9
Conventional	146	20.9	17.1	114	4.98	10.9
B						
SFE	179	21.2	25.4	291	3.86	11.0
Conventional	169	21.4	19.2	145	3.02	3.29
C						
SFE	198	20.9	21.5	195	11.1	ND[c]
Conventional	201	28.2	21.4	165	9.59	2.33
D						
SFE	272	28.1	13.9	188	2.57	ND
Conventional	255	36.0	12.3	151	2.03	ND

[a] Prokopczyk et al.[16]
[b] Data determined by single extraction using internal standard.
[c] ND, not detected.

tive tract in adult males. Among a random sample of 2868 males in the Nile province, 32.3% were toombak dippers and an additional 9.2% smoked cigarettes and used toombak, while 11.9% smoked cigarettes only.[17] The incidence of cancer of the oral cavity among males in northern Sudan between 1967 and 1984 was 9.7/100,000,[18] which compares with a rate of 11.2 among white males in the U.S. during 1983 to 1987. Of the U.S. cases, 91.5% were cigarette smokers.[19] The residents of the northern Sudan are Moslems who do not consume alcoholic beverages; thus, we are dealing with a uniquely different population (compared with U.S. cases); 50 out of 62 cases with oral cancer (interviewed in 1988 at the Department of Oral Surgery at the University of Khartoum) had a history of toombak dipping in the absence of alcohol as an etiologic factor.[20]

Toombak is made from locally grown *Nicotiana rustica,* which has high nicotine and nornicotine content. Four parts of finely ground tobacco leaves are mixed with one part of natron powder to which water is added to give a sticky product. The preparation is kept for at least 2 h in a closed tin container before it is placed into the oral vestibule, usually between the lower lip and gingiva, for periods lasting from a few minutes to several hours. The first report on the high concentrations of nicotine and TSNA in toombak originates from the International Agency for Research on Cancer in Lyon, France (Table 2).[21] We also found high concentrations of TSNA in five samples of toombak, although not quite as high as reported by the Lyon group[16] (Table 2). The TSNA values are 100-fold higher than in U.S. or Swedish snuff.[22] The TSNA analyses of the saliva of Sudanese toombak dippers yield in general at least tenfold higher levels than are reported for the saliva of U.S. snuff dippers (Table 3).[17,22,23]

TABLE 2
Levels of Nicotine and Tobacco-Specific _N_-Nitrosamines in Snuff and Toombak[a]

Sample[b]		Nicotine (mg/g)	NNN (µg/g)	NNK (µg/g)	NAT (µg/g)	NAB (µg/g)	Ref.
U.S.							
A (6)	1980–92	17.1–23.4	6.4–26.5	0.5–4.65	9.8–44.0[d]		10
B (7)	1980–92	21.0–30.7	5.7–64.0	0.7–4.6	3.9–44.0[d]		
C (1)	1990	21.5	41.4	1.24	2.97[d]		
Sweden							
A (5)	1980–90	12.4–15.1	5.67–7.83	1.0–2.08	2.2–5.13[d]		10
B (5)	1980–90	12.5–18.1	4.0–7.95	0.61–1.51	1.4–4.43[d]		
C (5)	1980–90	11.3	5.24–8.94	1.40–1.85	2.4–5.50[d]		
Toombak							
A (5)	1990	32.2–102.4	830–3080	630–7870	66–290	40–2370	21
B (5)	1990	8.4–26.0	420–1550	1140–2,790	30–140	60–210	
C (4)	1990	16.5–22.8	490–960	1170–2270	20–80	20–220	
D (4)	1990	17.9–40.6	850–1800	620–3830	50–130	90–230	
E (2)	1990	26.4–26.6	780–970	1610–1680	20–40	80	
Toombak							
I (5)[e]	1993		241–369	188–362	21–42	14–43	16

[a] All values are based on dry weight.
[b] Number in parenthesis = number of samples analyzed.
[c] In 1992, brand A accounted for 41.6% of the U.S. snuff market and brand B for 31%.
[d] NAT contains 5 to 10% NAB.
[e] Samples also contain 1.4 to 20.7 µg of _iso_-NNAL and not detected to 22.9 µg of NNAL per gram tobacco.

TABLE 3
Levels of Tobacco-Specific _N_-Nitrosamines in the Saliva of Snuff and Toombak Dippers

Sample	Year	No. of samples	TSNA (ng/g saliva)				Ref.
			NNN	NNK	NAT	NAB	
Snuff							
U.S.	1981	12	5–420	2–201	7–470[a]		41
	1986	30	37–225	ND[c]–61	48–555[a]		42
Sweden	1988	4	3–140	ND–16	4–85		43
Toombak							
Sudan	1991	12[b]	582–21,000	63–6690	ND–471	46–1944	23
	1993	6	14.8–105.7	20–135	2.3–20.4	2.6–14.2	16

[a] NAT contains 5 to 10% NAB.
[b] Saliva samples (12) contain 52 to 3272 ng of NNAL per milliliter of saliva.
[c] ND, not detected.

Biomarker studies have shown that in toombak chewers the hemoglobin adducts of NNN and NNK are very high, as are the urinary metabolites of NNK, 4-(methylnitrosamino)-1-(3-pyridyl)-1-butanol (NNAL), and NNAL-glucuronides.[24] These data support the concept that TSNA are human carcinogens and that toombak is a human carcinogen. Educational prevention efforts are strongly indicated to curtail the toombak habit among the residents in the northern Sudan.

V. TOBACCO SMOKE

Recent years have brought significant refinements for the analysis of TSNA in tobacco smoke. The formation of cigarette mainstream smoke (MS) and sidestream smoke (SS) yields considerable amounts of TSNA in addition to volatile N-nitrosamines (VNA). For MS analysis, ten to 40 cigarettes have to be individually smoked; SS analysis can be done with five to ten cigarettes. Figure 4 summarizes the separation scheme for the determination of TSNA; N-nitroso-n-pentylpicolylamine (NPePicA) serves as an internal standard for TSNA (Figure 5). The recovery rate of the method is better than 90% and the reproducibility for an individual TSNA is ± 5%.

A few years ago the trapping of the TSNA on a Cambridge glass fiber filter was challenged because this method might lead to artifactual formation of TSNA.[25] To verify this, a gas wash bottle containing ascorbic acid in citrate buffer is placed between the mouthpiece of the cigarette and the Cambridge filter; this solution inhibits the arti-

Analysis of TSNA

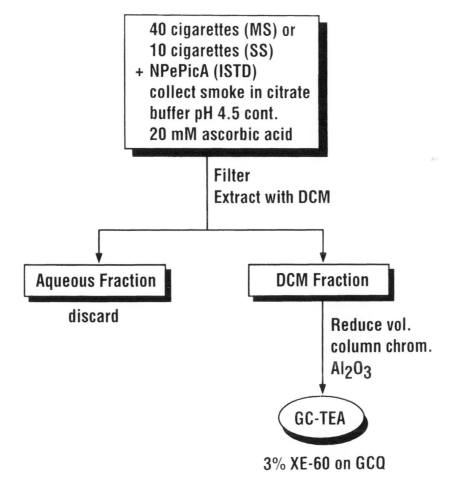

FIGURE 4. Analysis of TSNA in cigarette smoke.

GC-TEA Trace of TSNA in Cigarette Smoke

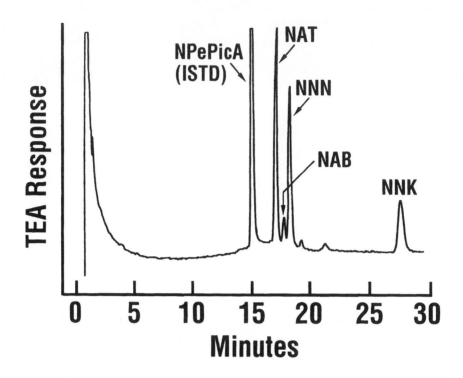

FIGURE 5. GC-TEA trace of TSNA in cigarette smoke.

TABLE 4
Tobacco-Specific Nitrosamines in Mainstream Smoke of Reference Cigarettes — Comparison of Trapping Methods (ng/cig.)

Cigarette	Trapping method	NNN	NAT	NAB	NNK	Total
KY 1R1	Gas wash bottle	16	19	ND[a]	13	48
	Filter	199	232	34	142	607
	Sum	215	251	34	155	655
	Filter direct	224	238	26	147	635
KY 2R1	Gas wash bottle	17	17	ND	12	46
	Filter	166	217	24	140	547
	Sum	183	234	24	152	593
	Filter direct	182	235	19	157	593
KY 2R1F	Gas wash bottle	11	12	ND	8	31
	Filter	216	243	34	148	641
	Sum	227	255	34	156	672
	Filter direct	224	219	34	135	612

[a] ND, not detected (below 1 ng/cig.).

128

factual formation of nitrosamines. Table 4 presents the data obtained for the individual TSNA in the smoke as trapped on the Cambridge filter with and without the inserted trapping solution. Clearly, we did not detect any difference in the data with these two techniques, confirming an earlier finding by our group.[26]

Table 5 lists data for TSNA in the MS of five prototypes of U.S. commercial cigarettes. These are cigarettes without filter tips, with filter tips, filter cigarettes with low-"tar" yields (<10 mg) and with ultralow-"tar" yields (<5 mg). Clearly, low-yield and ultralow-yield filter cigarettes show significantly reduced emissions of TSNA in MS when smoked using the standard FTC method.[27]

Data for TSNA in SS of the same prototype of cigarettes are given in Table 6. As expected, filter tips have no influence on the yields of TSNA in SS. However, the ultralow-yield filter cigarette delivers higher TSNA in SS than the majority of the other cigarettes. We assume that the tobacco of this ultralow-yield cigarette is especially rich in nitrate, the major precursor for the nitrosating species in the tobacco and in the smoke.[28] Remarkable are the same or higher yields of NNK than of NNN in SS. This observation

confirms an earlier report.[29] The relatively high yields of NNK in SS indicate that the pyrosynthesis of this TSNA is more favored during the smoldering of cigarettes when SS is generated than during puff drawing.

Table 7 presents data for TSNA in the MS of some foreign cigarettes. As reported earlier,[22] cigarettes made from dark tobacco and marketed in Canada, France, and Uruguay are rich in nitrate, and their smoke is rich in TSNA compared with cigarettes made from bright or blended tobaccos. The relatively high levels of TSNA in the smoke from cigarettes made in Poland, Russia, and Thailand parallel the high yields in "tar."

The data for the MS of cigarettes presented so far are generated by standardized machine-smoking conditions of one puff of 35-ml volume per minute with a puff duration of 2 s.[27] It is long known that smokers of low-yield cigarettes have the tendency to smoke more intensely to satisfy a craving for nicotine.[30,31] Model studies with cigarettes smoked at a rate of not one, but three to four puffs per minute and with puff volumes larger than 35-ml have demonstrated that not only the "tar" and nicotine yields are increased but also the yields of TSNA (Table 8).[28,32] Together, the higher puffing intensities by

TABLE 5
Tobacco-Specific Nitrosamines in Mainstream Smoke of Domestic Cigarettes (ng/cig.)

Cigarette	Type	NNN	NAT	NAB	NNK	Total
A	NF	278	236	30	156	700
B	NF	274	238	26	168	706
C	F	287	216	27	194	724
D	F	209	172	21	156	558
E	F, M	264	212	31	151	658
F	F, M	151	126	16	126	419
G	F, M	250	192	20	173	635
H	F, L	122	102	12	106	342
I	F, L	138	114	14	87	353
J	F, UL	40	37	4.5	17	98

Note: NF, nonfilter; F, filter; M, menthol; L, light; UL, ultralight.

TABLE 6
Tobacco-Specific Nitrosamines in Sidestream Smoke of Domestic Cigarettes (ng/cig.)

Cigarette	Type	NNN	NAT	NAB	NNK	Total
A	NF	170	105	20	241	536
B	NF	305	166	40	468	979
C	F	200	124	16	330	670
D	F	191	119	19	312	641
E	F, M	213	127	20	240	600
F	F, M	227	159	26	302	714
G	F, M	238	132	24	303	697
H	F, L	189	115	18	321	643
I	F, L	214	132	18	216	580
J	F, UL	330	221	41	352	944

Note: F, filter; NF, nonfilter; M, menthol; L, light; UL, ultralight.

TABLE 7
Tobacco-Specific Nitrosamines in Mainstream Smoke of Foreign Cigarettes (ng/cig.)

Country	Brand	Type	NNN	NAT	NAB	NNK	Total
Brazil	A	F	90	98	10	70	268
	B	F	92	107	15	90	304
Canada	A	F[a]	306	100	23	220	649
	B	F, M	28	54	TR	59	141
	C	F[b]	28	50	TR	52	130
France	A	NF[a]	675	250	54	306	1285
Germany	A	F	96	85	8.5	78	268
	C20	F	130	108	12	68	318
Japan	A	F[b]	122	105	10.5	65	303
	A	F[b], L	103	79	9.0	51	242
Poland	A	F	322	234	32	181	769
Russia	A	NF	460	206	36	42	744
	A	F	415	194	36	41	686
Switzerland	A	F, UL	56	50	12	30	148
Thailand	A	F[a]	730	430	53	369	1582
	B	F	40	43	6.0	45	134
Uruguay	A	NF[a]	230	218	24	204	676

Note: F, filter; NF, nonfilter; M, menthol; L, light; UL, ultra-light; TR, trace (below 1 ng/cig.)

[a] Dark tobacco.
[b] Charcoal filter.

smokers of low-nicotine cigarettes, deeper inhalation, and higher yields of the carcinogenic TSNA in the smoke have been considered to be a major contributor to the sharp rise in adenocarcinoma of the lung among cigarette smokers.[33,34]

TABLE 8
Nicotine, TSNA, and BaP in Mainstream Smoke[a]

Cigarette	Puff (ml)	TPM	"Tar" (mg/cig.)	Nic	NAT	NAB	NNN (ng/cig.)	NNK	Total TSNA	BaP
A										
NF, SP, 85 mm	25	25.7	22.8	1.41	131	24	118	64	337	43.5
FTC tar 24; nic 1.5	30	28.3	23.7	1.36	134	16	131	74	356	44.4
Ventilation: N/A	35	26.8	23.6	1.37	190	24	177	101	492	23.0
Butt length: 23 mm	40	34.9	29.8	1.69	173	24	164	97	458	34.2
Avg. wt: 1.1136 g	45	39.7	33.9	1.74	129	18	124	79	349	41.0
B										
F, SP, 85 mm	25	17.7	14.7	0.84	136	11	125	59	332	
FTC tar 17; nic 1.1	30	19.2	16.6	0.88	140	11	131	62	344	
Ventilation: 6.1%	35	23.9	19.0	0.95	167	12	162	75	417	
Butt length: 28 mm	40	26.7	19.8	1.02	140	10	132	75	357	
Avg. wt: 0.9731 g	45	28.7	22.0	1.07	129	11	135	78	347	
C										
F, SP, 85 mm	25	7.4	6.6	0.47	74	ND[b]	72	37	183	
FTC tar 8; nic 0.6	30	8.5	7.5	0.44	77	ND	77	40	194	
Ventilation: 35.3%	35	9.9	8.6	0.52	91	10	81	48	230	
Butt length: 35 mm	40	12.6	11.4	0.61	96	11	88	49	244	
Avg. wt: 0.9260 g	45	14.6	13.0	0.63	91	ND	89	49	229	
D										
F, SP, 85 mm	25	7.7	7.1	0.04	37	6	24	25	93	
FTC tar 7.6; nic 0.03	30	9.2	8.6	0.04	46	8	31	31	116	
Ventilation: 26.6%	35	11.2	10.2	0.04	50	9	34	36	129	
Butt length: 35 mm	40	12.0	10.6	0.05	55	9	36	39	138	
Avg. wt: 0.8855 g	45	13.2	11.6	0.05	58	9	40	42	149	
E										
F, SP, 85 mm	25	0.9	0.8	0.06	12	2	10	5	28	2.6
FTC tar 1; nic 0.1	30	1.2	0.9	0.08	15	2	11	5	34	3.8
Ventilation: 73.3%	35	2.0	1.5	0.11	21	3	17	8	49	5.4
Butt length: 33 mm	40	2.2	1.8	0.14	26	5	23	10	64	6.4
Avg. wt: 0.8045 g	45	2.4	2.1	0.16	30	4	26	12	72	9.0

TABLE 8 (continued)
Nicotine, TSNA, and BaP in Mainstream Smoke[a]

Cigarette	Puff (ml)	TPM	"Tar" (mg/cig.)	Nic	NAT	NAB	NNN (ng/cig.)	NNK	Total TSNA	BaP
F, SP, 85 mm	25	1.0	1.0	0.07	6	1	6	3	16	
FTC tar 1; nic 0.1	30	1.4	1.3	0.10	8	2	8	4	22	
Ventilation: 76.8%	35	1.7	1.3	0.14	14	2	14	6	37	
Butt length: 34 mm	40	2.5	2.0	0.18	16	3	15	6	41	
Avg. wt: 0.7619 g	45	3.2	3.0	0.20	21	4	21	9	54	

[a] Filter cigarettes smoked with open air vents (Djordjevic et al.[28]).

[b] ND, not detected.

VI. TSNA IN INDOOR AIR

Since 1980, a number of epidemiological studies have incriminated involuntary smoking as a lung cancer risk.[35,36] The *N*-nitrosamines derived from nicotine are the only known tobacco-specific carcinogens in indoor air that is polluted by environmental tobacco smoke (ETS). Therefore, we developed a highly sensitive method for the determination of TSNA, based on filtration of the ETS through Cambridge filters that were treated with potassium bisulfite. The trapped particulates were extracted, the TSNA enriched by chromatography, and the TSNA concentrate analyzed by GC-TEA. Figure 6 presents a chromatogram of the TSNA concentrate obtained from ETS pollutants collected in a bar. Table 9 summarizes findings from the analysis of indoor air sampled at ten different locations.[37] As in the case of SS, ETS contains higher amounts of NNK than of NNN, primarily because SS is the major contributor to ETS. In general, these TSNA data for ETS are comparable with those reported by Klus et al.;[38,39] however, the TSNA values for ETS of bar 1 (Table 9) are exceptionally high. In a biomarker study, nonsmokers were exposed to high concentrations of ETS in a test laboratory. Urine samples of these volunteers were subsequently analyzed for the metabolites of NNK, NNAL, and NNAL-glucuronide. The results of this study clearly demonstrate that NNK in ETS was retained, absorbed, and metabolized by the nonsmokers.[40] These findings support the concept that nonsmokers exposed to ETS have an increased risk for lung cancer.

It is the ultimate goal of the TSNA analyses of ETS to develop a marker method for estimating the contribution of ETS to the various settings of indoor pollution.

VII. SUMMARY

During the past 4 years, several new observations have been made on the formation of TSNA and their occurrence in smokeless tobacco, and MS, and SS of American and foreign cigarettes. Analysis of TSNA in oral snuff that had been incubated with saliva indicated greater presence of the more polar TSNA than was observed in analyses of extracts obtained by conventional organic solvent extraction. When snuff was extracted by means of supercritical fluid extraction with carbon dioxide containing 10% methanol, analysis of this material confirmed that the extraction with organic solvents had been incomplete. Storage of snuff at room temperature for 4 weeks leads to a reduction of

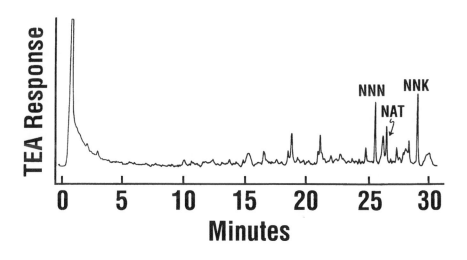

FIGURE 6. Gas chromatogram of TSNA found in indoor air.

TABLE 9
TSNA in Indoor Air (pg/l)

Site	Approx. # of cigarettes smoked	Collection time (h)	Flow rate (l/min)	NNN	NAT	NNK
Bar 1	25–35	3	3.2	22.8	9.2	23.8
Bar 2	10–15	3	3.2	8.3	6.2	9.6
Bar 3	10–15	3	3.2	4.3	3.7	11.3
Restaurant 1[a]	25–30	6	2.15	1.8	1.5	1.4
Restaurant 2[a]	40–50	8	2.1	ND[c]	ND	3.3
Car[b]	13	3.3	2.15	5.7	9.5	29.3
Train 1	50–60	5.5	3.3	ND	ND	4.9
Train 2	50–60	6	3.3	ND	ND	5.2
Office	25	6.5	3.3	ND	ND	26.1
Smoker's home	30	3.5	3.3	ND	ND	1.9

Note: Inhalation per 3 h (ng): NNN, 3.2–41; NNK, 2.5–43 (assuming a respiratory rate of 10 l/min). NNN, *N'*-nitrosonornicotine; NAT, *N*-nitrosoanatabine; NNK, 4-(methylnitrosamino)-1-(3-pyridyl)-1-butanone.

[a] Smoking section.
[b] Windows partially open.
[c] ND, not detected.

From Brunnemann, K. D., Cox, J. E., and Hoffmann, D., *Carcinogenesis*, 13, 2415, 1992. With permission.

nitrate to nitrite and, subsequently, to significant increases of TSNA due to nitrosation reactions. This explains, at least partially, why such remarkable variations in nitrite and TSNA content were found in the analyses of given snuff brands that were purchased in various regions in the U.S.

Epidemiological studies in the northern Sudan showed a high risk for oral cancer for users of toombak, a home-made oral snuff. Toombak contains 100-fold higher levels of TSNA than commercial snuff in the U.S. and Sweden. The TSNA content in the saliva of toombak dippers is at least ten times higher than that reported in the saliva of dippers of commercial snuff. Biomarker studies have shown corresponding high levels of hemoglobin adducts with metabolites of NNN and NNK as well as for urinary metabolites of NNK. These data supported the epidemiological findings.

The analyses of the MS of U.S. and foreign cigarettes smoked under FTC conditions revealed comparable data for the smoke of nonfilter cigarettes and filter cigarettes except in the case of low- and ultralow-yield cigarettes, which showed reduced TSNA yields. The MS of cigarettes made from Burley or dark tobacco is exceptionally high in TSNA, primarily because of the high nitrate content of those tobacco types. Taking puffs of larger volume and drawing puffs more frequently, practices observed among most smokers of cigarettes with low nicotine yield, results in high TSNA values in the MS. The formation of the lung carcinogen NNK is favored during the smoldering of cigarettes, between puffs, when SS is generated. Consequently, in most samples from indoor air polluted with ETS, the highest concentration of an individual TSNA is that of NNK. When nonsmokers had remained for up to 2 h in a test laboratory with high ETS pollution, they excreted measurable amounts of NNK metabolites in the urine, indicative of the absorption of TSNA.

ACKNOWLEDGMENTS

The authors greatly appreciate the technical support of Jonathan E. Cox, Yin Liu, and Jingrun Fan as well as the editorial assistance of Jennifer Johnting. Our studies are supported by grant CA-29580 from the U.S. National Cancer Institute.

REFERENCES

1. **Hoffmann, D., Rivenson, A., Murphy, S. E., Chung, F.-L., Amin, S., and Hecht, S. S.,** Cigarette smoking and adenocarcinoma of the lung: the relevance of nicotine-derived *N*-nitrosamines, *J. Smoking Relat. Disord.*, 4, 165, 1993.

2. **Hecht, S. S., Chen, C.-H. B., Ornaf, R. M., Jacobs, E., Adams, J. D., and Hoffmann, D.,** Reaction of nicotine and sodium nitrite: formation of nitrosamines and fragmentation of the pyrrolidine ring, *J. Org. Chem.*, 43, 72, 1978.

3. **Caldwell, W. S., Greene, J. H., Plowchalk, D. R., and deBethizy, J. D.,** The nitrosation of nicotine. A kinetic study, *Chem. Res. Toxicol.*, 4, 513, 1991.

4. **Smith, P. A. S. and Loeppky, R. N.,** Nitrosative cleavage of tertiary amines, *J. Am. Chem. Soc.*, 89, 1147, 1967.

5. **Mirvish, S. S., Sams, J., and Hecht, S. S.,** Kinetics of nornicotine and anabasine nitrosation in relation to N'-nitrosonornicotine occurrence in tobacco and to tobacco-induced cancer, *J. Natl. Cancer Inst.*, 59, 1211, 1977.

6. **Burton, H. R., Bush, L. P., and Djordjevic, M. V.,** Influence of temperature and humidity on the accumulation of tobacco-specific nitrosamines in stored burley tobacco, *J. Agric. Food Chem.*, 37, 1725, 1989.

7. **Andersen, R. A., Burton, H. R., Fleming, P. D., and Hamilton-Kemp, T. R.,** Effect of storage conditions on nitrosated, aceylated, and oxidized pyridine alkaloid derivatives in smokeless tobacco products, *Cancer Res.*, 49, 5895, 1989.

8. **Andersen, R. A., Fleming, P. D., Burton, H. R., Hamilton-Kemp, T. R., Hildebrand, D. T., and Sutton, T. G.,** Nitrosated, aceylated, and oxidized pyridine alkaloids and their derivatives in air- and flue-cured KY71 dark tobacco during prolonged storage; effects of temperature and moisture, *Tobacco Sci.*, 34, 50, 1990.

9. **Andersen, R. A., Fleming, P. D., Burton, H. R., Hamilton-Kemp, T. R., and Sutton, T. G.,** Nitrosated, aceylated and oxidized pyridine alkaloids during storage of smokeless tobacco: effects of moisture, temperature and their interactions, *J. Agric. Food Chem.*, 39, 1280, 1991.

10. **Djordjevic, M. V., Fan, J., Bush, L. P., Brunnemann, K. D., and Hoffmann, D.,** Effects of storage conditions on levels of tobacco-specific *N*-nitrosamines and *N*-nitrosamino acids in U.S. moist snuff, *J. Agric. Food. Chem.*, 41, 1790, 1993.

11. **Hoffmann, D., Djordjevic, M. V., Fan, J., Zang, E., Glynn, T., and Connolly, G. N.,** Five leading U.S. commercial brands of moist snuff in 1994. Assessment of carcinogenic N-nitrosamines, *J. Natl. Cancer Inst.*, 87, 1862, 1995.

12. **Djordjevic, M. V., Brunnemann, K. D., and Hoffmann, D.,** The need for regulation of carcinogenic *N*-nitrosamines in oral snuff. *Food Chem. Toxicol.*, 31, 497, 1993.

13. **Bush, L. P., Burton, H., Dye, N., and Nicholas, N.,** Post-harvest treatment effects on TSNA accumulation, Abstr. 48th Tobacco Chem. Res. Conf., Greensboro, NC, 1994, 41–42.

14. **Prokopczyk, B., Wu, M., Cox, J. E., and Hoffmann, D.,** Bioavalability of tobacco-specific *N*-nitrosamines to the snuff dipper, *Carcinogenesis*, 13, 863, 1992.

15. **Prokopczyk, B., Hoffmann, D., Cox, J. E., Djordjevic, M. V., and Brunnemann, K. D.,** Supercritical fluid extraction in the determination of tobacco-specific *N*-nitrosamines in smokeless tobacco, *Chem. Res. Toxicol.*, 5, 336, 1992.

16. **Prokopczyk, B., Wu, M., Cox, J. E., Amin, S., Desai, D., Idris, A. M., and Hoffmann, D.,** Improved methodology for the quantitative assessment of tobacco-specific N-nitrosamines in tobacco by supercritical fluid extraction. *J. Agric. Food Chem.,* 43, 916, 1995.

17. **Idris, A. M., Prokopczyk, B., and Hoffmann, D.,** Toombak: a major risk factor for cancer of the oral cavity in Sudan, *Prev. Med.,* 23, 832, 1994.

18. **Hidaytalla, A.,** Geographic and Ethnic Distribution of Malignant Neoplasia in Sudan, Ph.D. thesis. Sudan, University of Khartoum, 1988.

19. **Shopland, D. R., Eyre, H.-J., and Pechacek, T. F.,** Smoking-attributable cancer mortality in 1991: is lung cancer now the leading cause of death among smokers in the United States?, *J. Natl. Cancer Inst.,* 83, 1142, 1991.

20. **El-beshir, E. I., Abeen, H. A., Idris, A. M., and Abbas, K.,** Snuff dipping and oral cancer in Sudan: a retrospective study. *Br. J. Oral. Maxillofac. Surg.,* 27, 243, 1989.

21. **Idris, A. M., Nair, J., Ohshima, H., Friesen, M., Brouet, I., Faustman, E. M., and Bartsch, H.,** Unusually high levels of carcinogenic tobacco-specific nitrosamines in Sudan snuff (toombak), *Carcinogenesis,* 12, 1115, 1991.

22. **Hoffmann, D., Brunnemann, K. D., Prokopczyk, B., and Djordjevic, M. V.,** Tobacco-specific N-nitrosamines and Areca-derived N-nitrosamines: chemistry, biochemistry, carcinogenicity and relevance to humans, *J. Toxicol. Environ. Health,* 41, 1, 1994.

23. **Idris, A. M., Nair, J., Ohshima, H., Friesen, M., Brouet, I., Faustman, E. M., and Bartsch, H.,** Carcinogenic tobacco-specific nitrosamines are present at unusually high levels in the saliva of oral snuff users in Sudan, *Carcinogenesis,* 13, 1001, 1992.

24. **Murphy, S. E., Carmella, S. G., Idris, A. M., and Hoffmann, D.,** Uptake and metabolism of carcinogenic levels of tobacco-specific nitrosamines by Sudanese snuff dippers, *Cancer Epidemiol. Biomarkers Prev.,* 3, 423, 1994.

25. **Caldwell, W. S. and Conner, J. M.,** Artifact formation during trapping. An improved method for the determination of N-nitrosamines in cigarette smoke, in 43rd Tobacco Chem. Res. Conf., Richmond, Virginia, Abstr. 45, 1989.

26. **Djordjevic, M. V., Sigountos, C. W., Brunnemann, K. D., and Hoffmann, D.,** Formation of 4-(methylnitrosamino)-4-(3-pyridyl)butyric acid *in vitro* and in mainstream cigarette smoke, *J. Agric. Food Chem.,* 39, 209, 1991.

27. **Pillsbury, H. C., Bright, C. C., O'Connor, K. J., and Irish, F. W.,** Tar and nicotine in cigarette smoke, *J. Assoc. Off. Anal. Chem.,* 52, 458, 1969.

28. **Djordjevic, M. V., Sigountos, C. W., Brunnemann, K. D., and Hoffmann, D.,** Tobacco-specific nitrosamine delivery in mainstream smoke of high- and low-yield cigarettes smoked with varying puff volume, in Proc. CORESTA Symp., Kallithea, Greece, 1990, 54–62.

29. **Adams, J. D., O'Mara-Adams, K. J., and Hoffmann, D.,** Toxic and carcinogenic agents in undiluted mainstream and sidestream smoke of different types of cigarettes, *Carcinogenesis,* 8, 729, 1987.

30. **U.S. Surgeon General,** The Health Consequences of Smoking. Nicotine Addiction, DHHS (CDC)86-8406, Rockville, MD, 1988.

31. **Benowitz, N. L. and Henningfield, J. E.,** Establishing a nicotine threshold for addiction, *N. Engl. J. Med.,* 331, 123, 1994.

32. **Fischer, S., Spiegelhalder, B., and Preussmann, R.,** Influence of smoking parameters on the delivery of tobacco-specific nitrosamines in cigarette smoke. A contribution to relative risk evaluation, *Carcinogenesis,* 10, 1059, 1989.

33. **Devesa, S. S., Shaw, G. L., and Blot, W. J.,** Changing patterns of lung cancer incidence by histological type, *Cancer Epidemiol. Biomarkers Prev.,* 1, 29, 1991.

34. **Wynder, E.L. and Hoffmann, D.,** Smoking and lung cancer: scientific challenges and opportunities, *Cancer Res.,* 54, 5284, 1994.

35. **U.S. Surgeon General,** The Health Consequences of Involuntary Smoking, DHHS Publ. No. (CDC)87-8398, 1986.

36. **Fontham, E. T. H., Correa, P., Reynolds, P., Wu-Williams, A., Buffer, P. S., Greenberg, R. S., Chen, V. W., Alverman, T., Boyd, R., Austin, D. R., and Liff, J.** Environmental tobacco smoke and lung cancer in nonsmoking women. A multicenter study, *J. Am. Med. Assoc.*, 271, 1752, 1994.

37. **Brunnemann, K. D., Cox, J. E., and Hoffmann, D.,** Analysis of tobacco-specific *N*-nitrosamines in indoor air, *Carcinogenesis*, 13, 2415, 1992.

38. **Klus, H., Begutter, H., Ball, M., and Intorp, M.,** Environmental tobacco smoke in real life situations, in *Indoor Air '87, Vol. 2: Environmental Tobacco Smoke, Multicomponent Studies. Radon, Sick Buildings, Odours and Irritants, Hyperactivities, and Allergies*, Seifert, B., Esdorn, H., Fischer, M., Rüden, H., and Wegner, J., Eds., Institute for Water, Soil and Air Hygiene, Berlin, 1987, 137.

39. **Klus, H., Begutter, H., Ball, M., and Intorp, M.,** Environmental tobacco smoke in real life situations, Poster handout, 4th Int. Conf. on Indoor Air Quality and Climate, Berlin, 1987 (not published in Ref. 38).

40. **Hecht, S. S., Carmella, S. G., Murphy, S. E., Akerkar, S., Brunnemann, K. D., and Hoffmann, D.,** A tobacco-specific lung carcinogen in the urine of men exposed to cigarette smoke, *N. Engl. J. Med.*, 329, 1543, 1993.

41. **Hoffmann, D. and Adams, J. D.,** Carcinogenic tobacco-specific *N*-nitrosamines in snuff and in the saliva of snuff dippers, *Cancer Res.*, 41, 4305, 1981.

42. **Palladino, G., Adams, J. D., Brunnemann, K. D., Haley, N. J., and Hoffmann, D.,** Snuff dipping in college students: a clinical profile, *Mil. Med.*, 151, 342, 1986.

43. **Österdahl, B.-G. and Slorach, S.,** Tobacco-specific *N*-nitrosamines in the saliva of habitual male snuff dippers, *Food Addit. Contam.*, 5, 581, 1988.

Article 2

SYNTHESIS OF TOBACCO-SPECIFIC *N*-NITROSAMINES AND THEIR METABOLITES AND RESULTS OF RELATED BIOASSAYS

Critical Reviews in Toxicology, 26(2):139–147 (1996)

Synthesis of Tobacco-Specific *N*-Nitrosamines and Their Metabolites and Results of Related Bioassays

Shantu Amin, Dhimant Desai, Stephen S. Hecht, and Dietrich Hoffmann

American Health Foundation, Valhalla, NY 10595

ABSTRACT: Tobacco-specific *N*-nitrosamines (TSNA) are the most abundant, strong carcinogens in tobacco smoke. Seven TSNA have been identified in tobacco products: *N'*-nitrosonornicotine (NNN), *N'*-nitrosoanabasine (NAB), *N'*-nitrosoanatabine (NAT), 4-(methylnitrosamino)-1-(3-pyridyl)-1-butanone (NNK), 4-(methylnitrosamino)-1-(3-pyridyl)-1-butanol (NNAL), 4-(methylnitrosamino)-4-(3-pyridyl)-1-butanol (*iso*-NNAL), and 4-(methylnitrosamino)-4-3-pyridyl)butyric acid (*iso*-NNAC). The syntheses of these compounds are reviewed. The syntheses of ^{14}C- and ^{3}H-labeled NNK as well as metabolites of NNK and NNN are also discussed.

Comparative assays for lung tumorigenesis in female A/J mice were carried out for six of the TSNA and for two related compounds, *N*-nitrosodimethylamine (NDMA) and *N*-nitrosopyrrolidine (NPYR). They yielded the following ranking of potency: NDMA>NNK>NNAL>NPYR>NNN>NAB. *Iso*-NNAL and *iso*-NNAC were inactive. These results are also compared with previous assays of TSNA carcinogenicity in rats and hamsters.

KEY WORDS: synthesis, tobacco-specific *N*-nitrosamines, carcinogenicity, lung, oral cavity, pancreas, esophagus, metabolic activation, α-hydroxylation.

I. SYNTHESIS OF TSNA

N'-Nitrosonornicotine (NNN) was the first *N*-nitrosamine derived from the *Nicotiana* alkaloids to be identified in tobacco products.[1,2] Its synthesis was simple, namely, by nitrosation of nornicotine.[3] Similarly, the syntheses of *N'*-nitrosoanabasine (NAB) and *N'*-nitrosoanatabine (NAT) were accomplished by nitrosation of the corresponding secondary amines.[4,5] Model studies have shown that nitrosation of nicotine leads not only to NNN formation, but also to the opening of the pyrrolidine ring at the 1',2'-positions, yielding 4-(methylnitrosamino)-1-(3-pyridyl)-1-butanone (NNK), and the 1',5'-position, yielding 4-(methylnitrosamino)-4-(3-pyridyl)butanal (NNA; Figure 1).[6] The

presence of NAT, NAB, and NNK in tobacco and tobacco smoke has been established.[5] Because NNK and its metabolic reduction product 4-(methylnitrosamino)-1-(3-pyridyl)-1-butanol (NNAL) are present in tobacco products and were needed for bioassays,[7] we synthesized both compounds in gram amounts[8,9] and for biochemical studies also in ^{14}C-labeled and ^{3}H-labeled form (Figure 2).[10,11]

Tobacco also contains 4-(methylnitrosamino)-4-(3-pyridyl)-1-butanol (*iso*-NNAL), which is the reduction product of the aldehyde 4-(methylnitrosamino)-4-(3-pyridyl)-1-butanal (NNA). The oxidation product of NNA, namely, 4-(methylnitrosamino)-4-(3-pyridyl)butyric acid (*iso*-NNAC; Figure 1), is present as well. Both TSNAs were synthe-

1040-8444/96/$.50

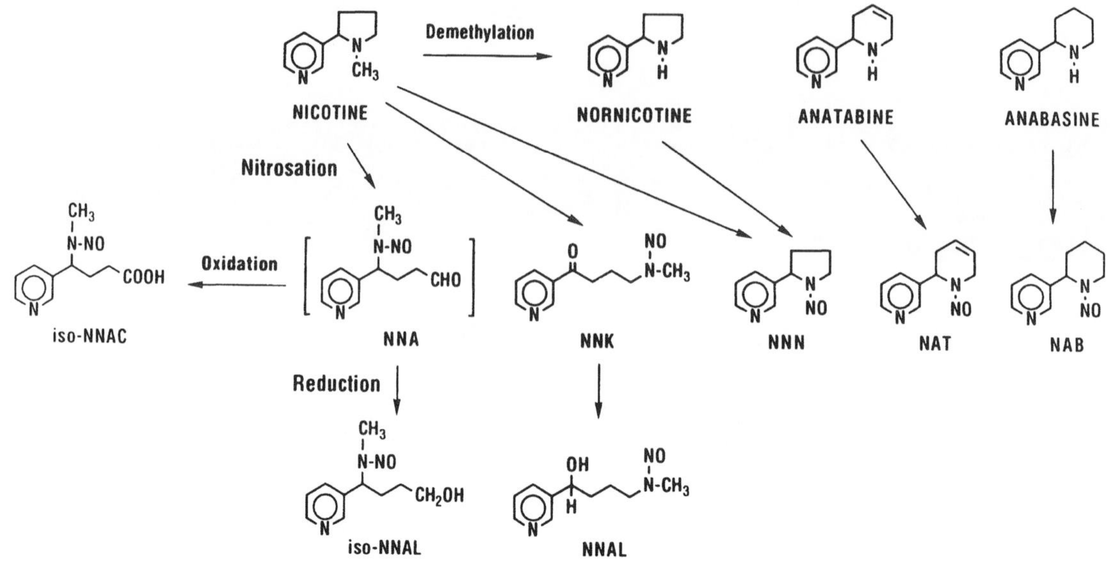

FIGURE 1. Formation of TSNA from the tobacco alkaloids nicotine, nornicotine, anatabine, and anabasine.

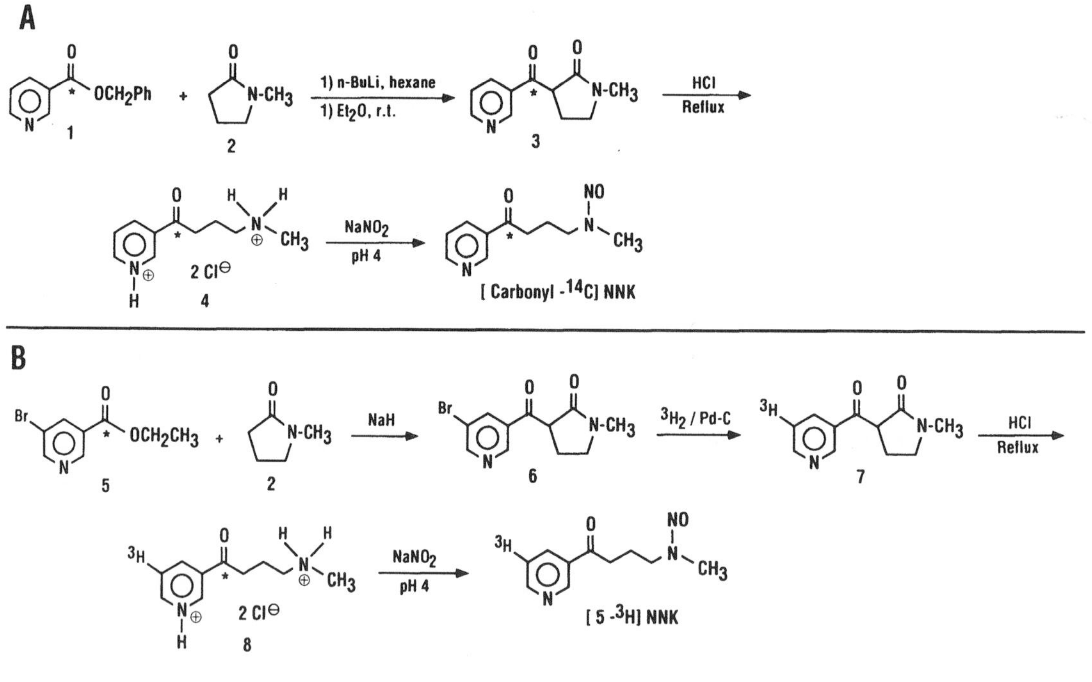

FIGURE 2. Synthesis of (A) [carbonyl-^{14}C]NNK and (B) [5-^{3}H]NNK, as described in References 10 and 11.

sized by us as reference compounds and, on a larger scale, for genotoxicity and carcinogenicity assays in rodents (Figure 3).[7,12] *Iso-*

NNAL and NNA were first prepared by reductive amination of 4-hydroxy-1-(3-pyridyl)-1-butanone (HPB), followed by

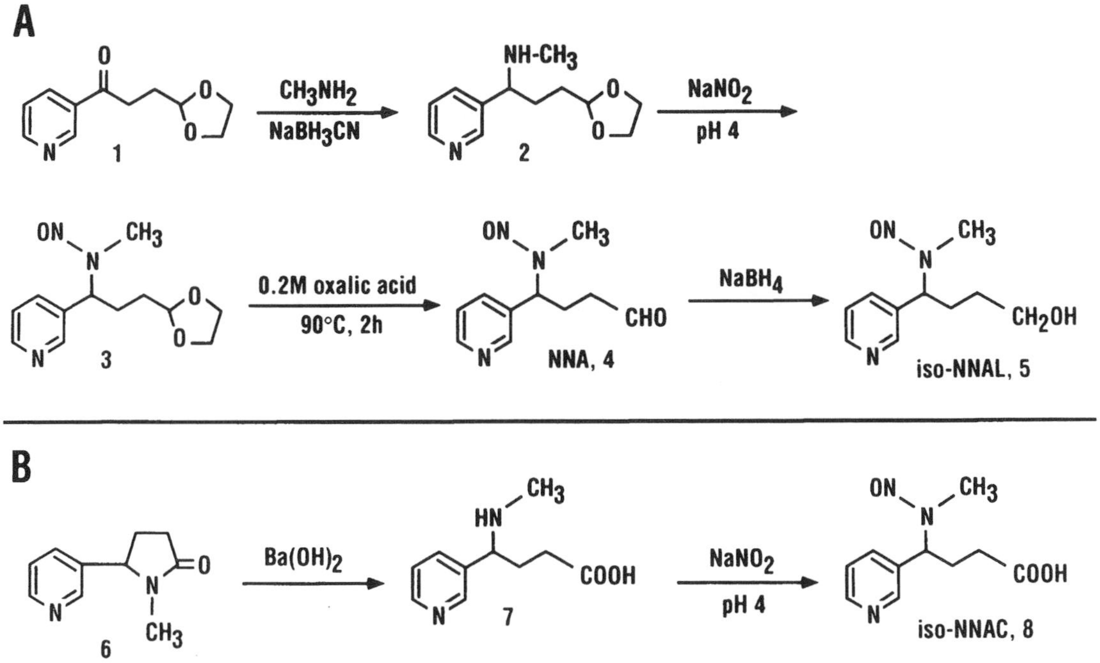

FIGURE 3. Synthesis of (A) NNA and *iso*-NNAL and (B) *iso*-NNAC.

nitrosation to give *iso*-NNAL, and by oxidation of this alcohol to the aldehyde NNA.[8] An improved synthesis is outlined in Figure 3A. The ketal **1** is prepared from potassium nicotinate and the Grignard reagent of 2-(2-bromoethyl)-1,3-dioxolane.[13] This ketal is the key intermediate for the preparation of NNA (**4**) and *iso*-NNAL (**5**), as illustrated. The synthesis of *iso*-NNAC is summarized in Figure 3B. Cotinine was hydrolyzed with Ba(OH)$_2$ and nitrosated at pH 4 to give *iso*-NNAC (**8**) in good yield.

II. SYNTHESIS OF METABOLITES OF TSNA

Four of the seven identified TSNA are procarcinogens that require metabolic activation by α-hydroxylation to exert carcinogenic activity.[14,15] The metabolic pathways of NNK and NNN, the two most carcinogenic TSNA, have been studied in some detail by our group. An overview of NNK and NNN metabolism is presented in Figure 4.[15]

All metabolites have been characterized by their spectral properties or by comparison to synthetic standards. The following metabolites were first synthesized in connection with these studies: racemic NNAL,[9] NNK-*N*-oxide (**1**),[9] NNN-*N*-oxide (**2**),[16] 3'- and 4'-OH-NNN (**4** and **5**),[16] NNAL-*N*-oxide (**6**),[17] 6-OH-NNK (**11**),[18] keto aldehyde **15**,[9] lactol **25**,[19] HPB (**26**),[8] and diol **27**.[9] As an example, the synthesis of 6-OH-NNK is illustrated in Figure 5.[18]

The key intermediate in this synthesis is the benzyl ether-protected lactam, which on deprotection by mild hydrogenolysis gives the hydroxy lactam, **5**. Hydrolysis of **5** with 6 *N* HCl, followed by nitrosation at pH 4 gives 6-OH-NNK in good yield. Several metabolites that are formed from nicotine had been prepared previously. These include norcotinine (**3**), keto acid **21**, hydroxy acid **28**, and lactone **29**.[20,21] High-pressure liquid chromatography (HPLC) separation of several known and potential metabolites of NNK is illustrated in Figure 6.

141

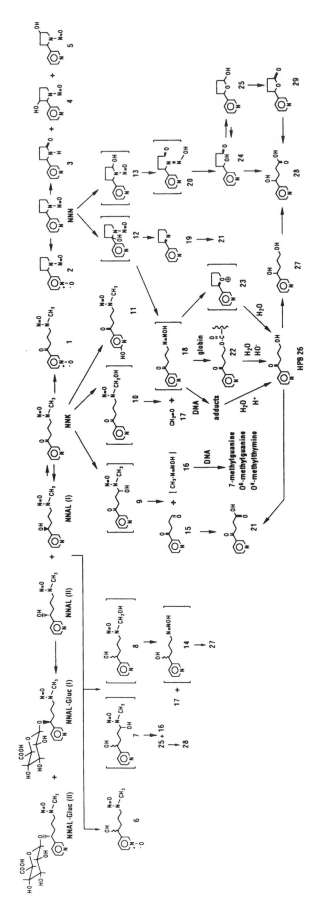

FIGURE 4. Metabolic fate of NNK and NNN in rodents and primates.

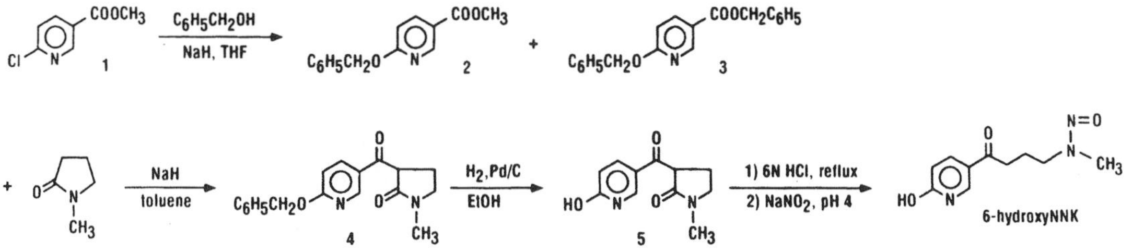

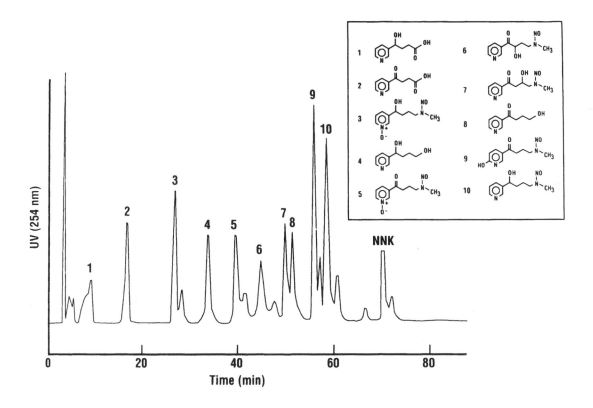

FIGURE 5. Synthesis of 6-hydroxyNNK, as described in Reference 18.

FIGURE 6. HPLC separation of ten known or potential metabolites of NNK. A 4.5 mm × 25 cm Whatman 5μ C-18 Partisphere column was used. Solvent A is 20 m*M* sodium phosphate buffer, pH 7.0, and solvent B is methanol. The program is to 35% B in 70 min with a 15-min hold at 15 min and a flow rate of 1 ml/min.

III. COMPARATIVE TUMORIGENICITY OF SOME TSNA AND RELATED NITROSAMINES IN A/J MICE

The strain A/J mouse lung adenoma assay has evolved as a suitable model assay for comparative evaluation of tumorigenic activities of *N*-nitrosamines that occur in tobacco products. Our comparative bioassay of eight *N*-nitrosamines (Table 1) was done with 440 female A/J mice, 6 to 8 weeks of age (Jackson Laboratories, Bar Harbor, ME) ranging from 18.0 ± 2.0 g in body weight.[22] These mice were housed in groups of five in solid-bottom polycarbonate cages with hardwood bedding at $20 \pm 2°C$ and $50 \pm 10\%$ relative humidity in a 12-h light/dark cycle.

TABLE 1
Tumors Induced in Female A/J Mice by TSNA and Related Nitrosamines

Group #	N-Nitrosamine		No. of Mice	Total Dose		Lung Adenomas		Other Tumors
				umol/ mouse	mmol/ kg	% Mice with tumors	Tumors per mouse±S.D.	
1		NDMA	30	5.0	0.25	100[a]	23.7± 8.9	1 Liver
2		NDMA	20	20.0	1.09	100[a]	38.7± 9.7	5 Liver[b]
3		NNK	30	5.0	0.25	76.7	1.6± 1.2	
4		NNK	20	20.0	1.01	100[a]	9.2± 6.3	1 Liver
5		NNAL	30	10.0	0.50	73.3	1.5± 1.4	
6		NNAL	20	50.0	2.52	100	9.7± 6.4	
7		NPYR	30	20.0	1.00	86.7	2.9± 1.8	
8		NPYR	30	100.0	5.24	93.3	3.6± 2.3	1 Liver
9		NNN	30	40.0	2.00	43.3	0.7± 1.0	
10		NNN	30	200.0	10.4	80.0[a]	2.3± 2.1	1 Liver
11		NAB	31	100.0	5.38	90.3[a]	1.8± 1.1	
12		Iso-NNAL	30	200.0	10.0	30.0[a]	0.43± 0.12	
13		Iso-NNAC	30	200.0	10.5	26.7	0.33± 0.61	
14	Saline	Neg. Control	30	-	-	26.7	0.27± 0.58	1 Liver

[a]Mice with lung adenocarcinoma: group 1,4/30; group 2, 2/20; groups 10,11 & 12, 1 each

[b]Three mice had liver carcinoma

NIH-07 diet and tapwater were given *ad lib*. The test solutions were freshly prepared each week and were administered by i.p. injection of 0.1 ml, three times weekly for 7 weeks. The mice were then observed for 30 weeks. Body weights were determined weekly for the first 4 weeks and then once every 4 weeks. Thirty weeks after the last injection, the mice were killed by cervical dislocation. Lung adenomas were counted. Lung tumor multiplicity data were subjected to an analysis of variance, nested model (cages were nested), followed by Scheffe's test for multiple comparison of means (pairwise).[23,24]

In the comparative bioassay in A/J mice there were no toxic effects, as indicated by the average weights of the animals throughout the bioassay, except for the positive control mice treated with NDMA at a total dose of 20 μmol. At 5 μmol per animal, NDMA was not toxic. The maximum tolerated dose of NAB was 100 μmol per mouse. Table 1 summarizes the results. According to the analysis of variance of tumor multiplicity, NDMA was the most powerful inducer of lung adenomas, followed by NNK, NNAL, NPYR, NNN, and NAB. *Iso*-NNAL and *iso*-NNAC were inactive.

In this bioassay, a total of 20 μmol of NNK per mouse induced 9.2 ± 6.3 tumors per mouse, which is consistent with earlier studies.[25,26] A dose of 200 μmol NNN per mouse induced 2.3 tumors per mouse, whereas 100 μmol of NPYR induced 3.6 tumors per mouse. These findings were also in line with earlier bioassay data.[25-27] In this assay, as in an earlier one, 200 μmol per mouse of *iso*-NNAC did not induce tumors in A/J mice.[28]

TSNA and related nitrosamines were also tested earlier in rats and in Syrian golden hamsters. Druckrey et al. had administered NDMA and NPYR to BD rats *per os*. Both compounds induced malignant tumors of the liver; however, NDMA was a much more active hepatocarcinogen than NPYR.[29] NNK was more carcinogenic than NNN in F-344 rats, inducing adenomas and adenocarcinoma of the lung, tumors of the nasal cavity, and a few liver tumors when administered by s.c. injection at total doses of 1, 3, and 9 mmol/kg. NNN induced nasal and esophageal tumors.[30] In another bioassay, NNK at a total dose of 3.4 mmol (9.8 mmol/kg) was more carcinogenic than NNN in F-344 rats.[31] When NNK and NNAL were given to F-344 rats in drinking water (5 ppm) at a total dose of 0.685 mmol/kg, both compounds induced primarily tumors of the lung and significant numbers of tumors of the exocrine pancreas.[32] The lung tumor assay in A/J mice has proven to be suitable for evaluating the potential carcinogenic activities of *N*-nitrosamines that occur in tobacco and tobacco smoke because the data obtained with this assay indicate relative carcinogenic potencies of TSNA similar to those observed in rats and hamsters. Furthermore, the assay in A/J mice can be concluded within 6 months and requires only 20 to 30 animals per group.

IV. FUTURE NEEDS

Recent studies at the American Health Foundation have shown that tobacco chewers and cigarette smokers excrete a significant portion of NNK in their urine as NNAL and its glucuronide (Figure 4). Two phenotypes recognized by different urinary ratios of NNAL glucuronide to NNAL may relate to lung cancer risk. NNAL is a known lung carcinogen and the glucuronide is expected to be a detoxification product. However, bioassays are required to confirm this. The results of these biomarker studies require that we determine the absolute configurations of the two enantiomeric forms of NNAL, as well as the diastereomeric glucuronides, to enable further characterization of the forms that are present in the urine of tobacco chewers and smokers.

We anticipate a need for the synthesis of DNA adducts of the metabolically activated forms of NNN and NNK, both at the nucleoside level and incorporated into defined oligomers. These will be used for structural and mutagenicity studies. The foregoing gives a few examples of the required teamwork of organic synthetic chemists with biochemists and molecular biologists in research on the carcinogenic effects of nicotine-derived *N*-nitrosamines, an area of major public health interest.

ACKNOWLEDGMENTS

Our studies are supported by grants CA-29580, CA-44377, and NO1-CP-21115 from the U.S. National Cancer Institute.

REFERENCES

1. **Klus, H., and Kuhn, H.,** Die Bestimmung des Nornikotin-Nitrosamins im Rauch Kondensat Nornikotin-reicher Zigaretten, *Fachliche Mitt. Oesterr. Tabakregie,* 14, 251, 1973.

2. **Hoffmann, D., Hecht, S. S., Ornaf, R. M., and Wynder, E. L.,** N'-Nitrosonornicotine in tobacco, *Science* , 186, 265, 1974.

3. **Hu, M. W., Bondinell, W. E., and Hoffmann, D.,** Synthesis of carbon-14 labelled myosmine, nornicotine, and N'-nitrosonornicotine, *J. Labelled Compd.,* 10, 79, 1974.

4. **Boyland, E., Roe, F. J. C., Gorrod, J. W., and Mitchley, B. C. V.,** Carcinogenicity of nitrosoanabasine, a possible constituent of tobacco smoke, *Br. J. Cancer,* 18, 265, 1964.

5. **Hoffmann, D., Adams, J. D., Brunnemann, K. D., and Hecht, S. S.,** Assessment of tobacco-specific N-nitrosamines in tobacco products, *Cancer Res.,* 39, 2505, 1979.

6. **Hecht, S. S., Chen, C. B., Ornaf, R. M., Jacobs, E., Adams, J. D., and Hoffmann, D.,** Reaction of nicotine and sodium nitrite: formation of nitrosamines and fragmentation of the pyrrolidine ring, *J. Org. Chem.,* 43, 72, 1978.

7. **Hoffmann, D., Brunnemann, K. D., Prokopczyk, B., and Djordjevic, M. V.,** Tobacco-specific N-nitrosamines and areca-derived N-nitrosamines: chemistry, biochemistry, carcinogenicity, and relevance to humans, *J. Toxicol. Environ. Health,* 41, 1, 1994.

8. **Hecht, S. S., Chen, C.-H. B., Dong, M., Ornaf, R. M., and Hoffmann, D.,** Studies on non-volatile nitrosamines in tobacco, *Beitr. Tabakforsch.,* 9, 1, 1977.

9. **Hecht, S. S., Young, R., and Chen, C. B.,** Metabolism in the F344 rat of 4-(N-methyl-N-nitrosamino)-1-(3-pyridyl)-1-butanone, a tobacco-specific carcinogen, *Cancer Res.,* 40, 4144, 1980.

10. **Wiley, J. C., Chien, D. H. T., Nungesser, N. A., Lin, D., and Hecht, S. S.,** Synthesis of 4-(methylnitrosamino)-1-(3-pyridyl)-1-butanone, 4-(carbethoxynitrosamino)-1-(3-pyridyl)-1-butanone, and N'-nitrosonornicotine labeled with tritium in the pyridine ring, *J. Labelled. Compd.,* 25, 707, 1988.

11. **Castonguay, A. and Hecht, S. S.,** Synthesis of carbon-14 labeled 4-(methylnitrosamino)-1-(3-pyridyl)-1-butanone, *J. Labelled Compd.,* 22, 23, 1985.

12. **Williams, G. M., Mori, H., and McQueen, C. A.,** Structure-activity relationships in the rat hepatocyte DNA-repair test for 300 chemicals, *Mutat. Res.,* 221, 263, 1989.

13. **Abbaspour, A., Hecht, S. S., and Hoffmann, D.,** Synthesis of 5'-carboxy-N'-nitrosonornicotine and 5'-([^{14}C]carboxy)-N'-nitrosonornicotine. *J. Org. Chem.,* 52, 3474, 1987.

14. **Hecht, S. S. and Hoffmann, D.,** The relevance of tobacco-specific nitrosamines in human cancer, *Cancer Surv.,* 8, 273, 1989.

15. **Hecht, S. S., Carmella, S. G., Foiles, P. G., and Murphy, S. E.,** Biomarkers for human uptake and metabolic activation of tobacco-specific nitrosamines, *Cancer Res.,* 54, 1912s, 1994.

16. **Hecht, S. S., Chen, C. B., and Hoffmann, D.,** Metabolic β-hydroxylation and N-oxidation of N'-nitrosonornicotine, *J. Med. Chem.,* 23, 1175, 1980.

17. **Castonguay, A., Tjülve, H., Trushin, N., and Hecht, S. S.,** Perinatal metabolism of the tobacco-specific carcinogen 4-(methyl-nitrosamino)-1-(3-pyridyl)-1-butanone in C57BL mice, *J. Natl. Cancer Inst.,* 72, 1117, 1984.

18. **Desai, D., Kagan, S. S., Amin, S., Carmella, S. G., and Hecht, S. S.,** Identification of 4-(methylnitrosamino)-1-[3-(6-hydroxy-pyridyl)]-1-butanone as a urinary metabolite of 4-(methylnitrosamino)-1-(3-pyridyl)-1-butanone in rodents, *Chem. Res. Toxicol.,* 6, 794, 1993.

19. **Chen, C. B., Hecht, S. S., and Hoffmann, D.,** Metabolic α-hydroxylation of the tobacco-specific carcinogen N'-nitrosonornicotine, *Cancer Res.,* 38, 3639, 1978.

20. **McKennis, H., Jr., Schwarts, S. L., Turnbull, L. B., Tamaki, E., and Bowman, E. R.,** The metabolic formation of c-(3-pyridyl)-c-hydroxybutyric acid and its possible intermediary role in the mammalian metabolism of nicotine, *J. Biol. Chem.,* 239, 3981, 1964.

21. **McKennis, H., Jr., Turnbull, L. B., Bowman, E. R., and Wada, E.,** Demethylation of

cotinine *in vivo, J. Am. Chem. Soc.,* 81, 3951, 1959.

22. **Hoffmann, D., Djordjevic, M. V., Rivenson, A., Zang, E., Desai, D., and Amin, S.,** A study of tobacco carcinogenesis. LI. Relative potencies of tobacco-specific *N*-nitrosamines as inducers of lung tumors in A/J mice, *Cancer Lett.,* 71, 25, 1993.

23. **Colton, T. C.,** *Statistics in Medicine,* Little, Brown, Boston, MA, 1974.

24. **Scheffe, H.,** *The Analysis of Variance,* John Wiley & Sons, New York, 1959.

25. **Castonguay, A., Lin, D., Stoner, G. D., Radok, P., Furuya, K., Hecht, S. S., Schut, H. A. J., and Klaunig, J. E.,** Comparative carcinogenicity in A/J mice and metabolism by cultured mouse peripheral lung of *N'*-nitrosonornicotine, 4-(methylnitrosamino)-1-(3-pyridyl)-1-butanone, and their analogues, *Cancer Res.* 43, 1223, 1983.

26. **Hecht, S. S., Abbaspour, A., and Hoffmann, D. A.,** study of tobacco carcinogenesis. XLII. Bioassay in A/J mice of some structural analogues of tobacco-specific nitrosamines, *Cancer Lett.,* 42, 141, 1988.

27. **Hecht, S. S., Chen, C-H. B., Hirota, N., Ornaf, R. M., Tso, T. C., and Hoffmann, D.,** Tobacco-specific nitrosamines: formation from nicotine in vitro and during tobacco curing, and carcinogenicity in strain A/J mice, *J. Natl. Cancer Inst.,* 60, 819, 1989.

28. **Rivenson, A., Djordjevic, M. V., Amin, S., and Hoffmann, D.,** A study of tobacco carcinogenesis. XLIV. Bioassay in A/J mice for some *N*-nitrosamines. *Cancer Lett.,* 47, 111, 1989.

29. **Druckrey, H., Preussmann, R., Ivankovic, S., and Schmaehl, D.,** Organotrope carcinogene Wirkungen bei 65 verschiedenen *N*-Nitroso-Verbindungen an BD-Ratten, *Z. Krebsforsch.,* 69, 102, 1967.

30. **Hoffmann, D., Rivenson, A., Amin, S., and Hecht, S. S.,** A study of tobacco carcinogenesis. XXVII. Dose-response study of the carcinogenicity of tobacco-specific *N*-nitrosamines in F344 rats, *J. Cancer Res. Clin. Oncol.,* 108, 81, 1984.

31. **Hecht, S. S., Chen, C. B., Ohmori, T., and Hoffmann, D.,** A study of tobacco carcinogenesis. XIX. Comparative carcinogenicity in F344 rats of the tobacco-specific nitrosamines, *N'*-nitrosonornicotine and 4-(methylnitrosamino)-1-(3-pyridyl)-1-butanone, *Cancer Res.,* 40, 298, 1980.

32. **Rivenson, A., Hoffmann, D., Prokopczyk, B., Amin, S., and Hecht, S. S.,** A study of tobacco carcinogenesis. XLII. Induction of lung and exocrine pancreas tumors in F344 rats by tobacco-specific and Areca-derived *N*-nitrosamines, *Cancer Res.,* 48, 6912, 1988.

ENDOGENOUS FORMATION OF NITROSAMINES AND OXIDATIVE DNA-DAMAGING AGENTS IN TOBACCO USERS

Critical Reviews in Toxicology, 26(2):149–161 (1996)

Endogenous Formation of Nitrosamines and Oxidative DNA-Damaging Agents in Tobacco Users

J. Nair,[1] H. Ohshima,[2] U. J. Nair, and H. Bartsch[1,]*

[1]Division of Toxicology and Cancer Risk Factors, German Cancer Research Center, Heidelberg, Germany; [2]Unit of Endogenous Cancer Risk Factors, International Agency for Research on Cancer, Lyon, France

* To whom correspondence should be addressed at the German Cancer Research Center, Division 0325, P.O. Box 101949, D-69009 Heidelberg, Germany.

ABSTRACT: One-third of all cancers worldwide can be attributed to various tobacco habits. Both in tobacco smoke and smokeless tobacco, carcinogenic *N*-nitroso compounds (NOC) are implicated as DNA-damaging agents in cancers of the aerodigestive tract and the pancreas. The exposure from nitrosamines in certain types of tobacco use such as "toombak" in Sudan could be as high as a few milligrams per day. Using the *N*-nitrosoproline test, it has been shown that smoking contributes to endogenous nitrosation and likely increases NOC formation *in vivo*. Smokeless tobacco, most widely used in the form of chewing of betel quid (BQ) with tobacco, was shown to particularly enhance endogenous nitrosation in the oral cavity, a site where chewing habits are causally associated with cancer. Poor oral hygiene was found to contribute to the formation of nitrosamines in the oral cavity. The evidence so far accumulated demonstrates that tobacco habits increase endogenous NOC formation, thus adding to the burden of exposure by preformed carcinogenic NOC in tobacco products. In snuff dippers, the unexpected higher level of HPB released from hemoglobin, an exposure marker for carcinogenic tobacco-specific nitrosamines, has been attributed to the endogenous formation of these carcinogens. Recent studies have demonstrated that besides carcinogenic tobacco-specific nitrosamines, reactive oxygen species derived from BQ ingredients could also play a role in the etiology of oral cancer in chewers. Although the use of chemopreventive agents may block nitrosation reactions *in vivo* in tobacco users, cessation of tobacco habits is the only safe way for an efficient reduction of cancer risk, in view of the high exposure to other (preformed) tobacco-related carcinogens.

KEY WORDS: tobacco, nitrosamines, *N*-nitrosoproline, endogenous, reactive oxygen species.

I. INTRODUCTION

Tobacco habits such as smoking, snuff dipping, and chewing of tobacco alone or with betel quid (BQ) ingredients have been causally associated in man with malignancies of the upper aerodigestive tract, pancreas, and renal pelvis.[1,2] About one-third of all cancers worldwide can be attributed to various tobacco habits,[3,4] and hence could be preventable by the cessation of the habits. Tobacco smoke contains several known classes of carcinogens such as polycyclic aromatic hydrocarbons, volatile and tobacco-specific nitrosamines (TSNA), and aromatic amines,[5] whereas in unburnt tobacco, very high concentrations (up to milligrams per gram of product) of TSNA have been reported.[6-8] Based on rodent bioassays that demonstrated the carcinogenicity of TSNA[9,10] and epidemiological studies that have causally associated tobacco habits to human cancer,[1,2] it is strongly suggested that TSNA contribute to the causation of human neoplasms.[11] In addition to the preformed nitroso compounds present in tobacco and tobacco smoke, nitrosamines could also be formed endogenously from nitrosatable alkaloids such as nornicotine, anatabine, and anabasine (present in hundreds of milligrams per gram of tobacco), and from nitrosatable amines such as pyrrolidine. Evidence is also accumulating for the endogenous synthesis of nitrosamines from nitric oxide (NO)-mediated reactions that are generated during inflammatory processes via nitric oxide synthase.[12] In addition, nitrosation modifiers such as thiocyanate (in saliva) and aldehydes (in smoke) may catalyze the nitrosation process in the body. The formation of reactive oxygen species (ROS) has been demonstrated from BQ ingredients such as areca nut and catechu, which are used frequently in India and other countries from Micronesia.[13] Several experimental studies have demonstrated that ROS can lead to DNA-base damage such as 8-hydroxydeoxyguanosine (8OH-dG) and thymine glycol, which are implicated in mutagenesis and carcinogenesis.[14] The following article reviews the current evidence for the formation of nitroso compounds in the human body, following the use of tobacco by various habits and by nitrosation processes that may also be enhanced during chronic cellular inflammatory conditions via the formation of NO. The role of endogenous formation of ROS and derived DNA damage, possibly acting synergistically with TSNA in the etiology of oral cancer, is also discussed.

II. ENDOGENOUS NITROSATION IN TOBACCO SMOKERS

After publication of a noninvasive test for assessing endogenous nitrosation in humans, the N-nitrosoproline (NPRO) test,[15] several studies have examined whether the excretion of NPRO is increased in smokers in order to demonstrate the endogenous nitrosamine formation. Hoffmann and Brunnemann[16] first showed that smokers excreted 1.4 times more NPRO in their urine than did nonsmokers. Ingestion of 300 mg of proline resulted in a 3.3-fold higher excretion of NPRO in smokers when both groups were kept on the same diet. Ladd et al.[17] showed a 2.5-fold higher excretion of urinary NPRO in smokers when compared with nonsmokers after the subjects had ingested 500 mg of proline and beet juice containing the equivalent of 325 mg of nitrate. In addition to NPRO, other nitrosamino acids excreted in urine such as N-nitrososarcosine, N-nitrosothiazolidine-4-carboxylic acid (NTCA), and the cis and trans isomers of N-nitroso-2-methylthiazolidine-4-carboxylic acid (NMTCA) have also been used to estimate the endogenous formation of nitroso compounds in tobacco smokers. Bartsch et al.[18] reported a twofold increase in the excretion of urinary total nitrosamino acids in smoking healthy subjects and chronic atrophic gastritis patients when compared with nonsmokers. Excretion of NPRO and NTCA was measured in a 24-h urine test of a small number of subjects from India who were smokers of Western-type cigarettes and/or bidi (a native form of smoking tobacco). A pronounced increased formation of these nitrosamino acids was detected in cigarette and bidi smokers.[19] An enhanced excretion (in the order of twofold) of NTCA and NMTCA has also been reported in the smokers.[20]

The above studies demonstrate that tobacco smoking at least doubles the exposure to nitroso compounds in smokers (Figure 1). The major factors influencing endogenous

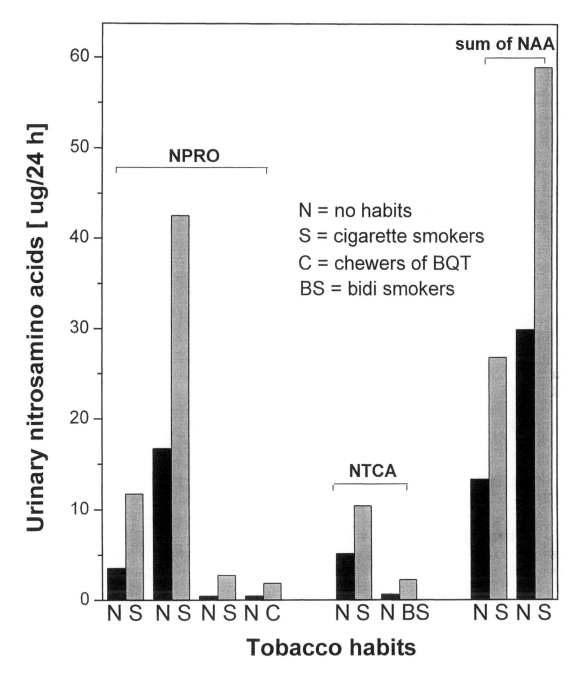

FIGURE 1. Nitrosamino acids (NAA) in urine of tobacco users NPRO, *N*-nitrosoproline; NTCA, *N*-nitrosothiazolidine-4-carboxylic acid. (Compiled and adapted from References 16 to 20.)

nitrosation reactions probably are the levels of nitrogen oxides (NO_x, nitrosating agents) in the smoke, salivary nitrate, and the thiocyanate metabolically formed from hydrogen cyanide. All are present in high concentrations (NO_x, up to a few hundred micro-

grams per smoked cigarette[5]), and smokers have higher thiocyanate levels in their saliva.[20] In addition, the formaldehyde and acetaldehyde present in tobacco smoke may further enhance the nitrosation reaction.[5] Nitrosatable secondary amines such as dimethylamine, pyrrolidine, and the alkaloids nornicotine, anabasine, and anatabine are present in tobacco smoke.[2]

III. *IN VITRO* NITROSATION OF TOBACCO AND BETEL QUID

Further evidence for the possible occurrence of endogenous formation of nitrosamines was obtained from *in vitro* studies by nitrosation of alkaloids present in tobacco and BQ. Incubation of chewing tobacco with saliva[21] and nitrosation under simulated gastric conditions[22] have revealed the formation of N'-nitrosonornicotine (NNN), N'-nitrosoanatabine (NAT), and N'-nitrosoanabasine (NAB). NNN, NAT, N-nitrosoguvacoline (NGCO), and N-nitrosoguvacine (NGCI) were shown to form when BQ with tobacco was incubated with physiological levels occurring in saliva of nitrite and thiocyanate at neutral and acidic pH.[23]

IV. ENDOGENOUS NITROSATION IN BETEL QUID CHEWERS

The urinary levels of NPRO and NTCA in chewers of BQ or BQ with tobacco (BQT) were found to be higher than in nonchewing subjects (Figure 1).[19] Because BQT chewing is strongly associated with oral cancer[1] and nitrosamines are the only major known carcinogens detected in unburnt tobacco, work has focused on assessing the burden of endogenously formed nitrosamines. Using a modified NPRO test, whereby 100 mg of proline was added to the BQ, and after 20 min, saliva was collected from each subject, it has been clearly shown that increased NPRO is formed while chewing BQT or BQ[24] (Figure 2), although the extent of increased nitrosation varied in individual subjects. Reduction of salivary NAT and NGCO levels in the same subject after chewing BQ/BQT together with ascorbic acid, which is a

known inhibitor of endogenous nitrosation, demonstrated that these nitroso compounds were formed during chewing. Further evidence for endogenous nitrosamine formation in the oral cavity was derived from the following three studies. (1) The areca nut-derived nitrosamines NGCO, NGCI, and 3-(nitrosomethylamino)propionitrile have been reported in the saliva of chewers of BQ or BQT,[23,25,26] which are formed only after nitrosation of areca alkaloids; they have not been reported to be present as preformed compounds in areca nut. (2) Osterdahl and Slorach[27] have shown that the total amount of TSNA measured in snuff after dipping was nearly the same as before dipping, in spite of the fact that high levels of TSNA were detected in the saliva collected during the dipping. A plausible explanation for this finding is that additional TSNA were formed during snuff dipping. (3) A higher level of 4-hydroxy-1-(3-pyridyl)-1-butanone (HPB)-hemoglobin adducts (a biomarker for TSNA exposure) was detected in snuff dippers when compared with cigarette smokers. As the exposure dose of TSNA (based on the average consumption and TSNA levels in these products) was similar in both groups, the higher amount of this HPB-Hb adduct has been attributed to the endogenous formation of TSNA in snuff dippers.[28]

Using NPRO as a probe, Nair et al.[29] demonstrated that endogenous nitrosation occurs at a significantly higher extent in subjects with poor oral hygiene as compared with those with good oral hygiene (Figure 3). This implies that after the bioavailability of nitrosatable amines (nornicotine, anatabine, and anabasine) from tobacco, there will be more formation of nitrosamines in subjects with poor oral hygiene if they chew tobacco. The enhanced endogenous nitrosation in subjects with poor oral hygiene may be due to the increased conversion of nitrate to nitrite, bacterial enzyme-mediated formation of nitrosamines, or both. Several bacterial strains isolated from vari-

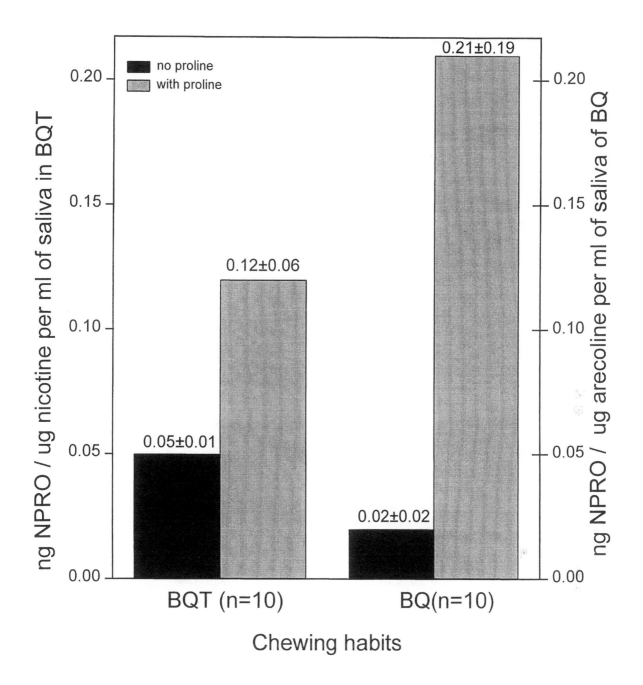

FIGURE 2. Formation of *N*-nitrosoproline in the oral cavity of chewers of betel quid (BQ) or BQ with tobacco (BQT). (Adapted from Nair, J., Nair, U. J., Ohshima, H., Bhide, S. V., and Bartsch, H., in *The Relevance of* N-*Nitroso Compounds in Human Cancer: Exposure and Mechanisms*, Bartsch, H., O'Neill, I. K., and Schulte-Herman, R., Eds., International Agency for Research on Cancer, Lyon, 1987, 465.)

ous human sources have been shown to catalyze the formation of nitrosamines,[30,31] and one nitrosating enzyme purified from bacteria had the characteristics of cytochrome cd1-nitrite reductase, generating NO during nitrite reduction.[32]

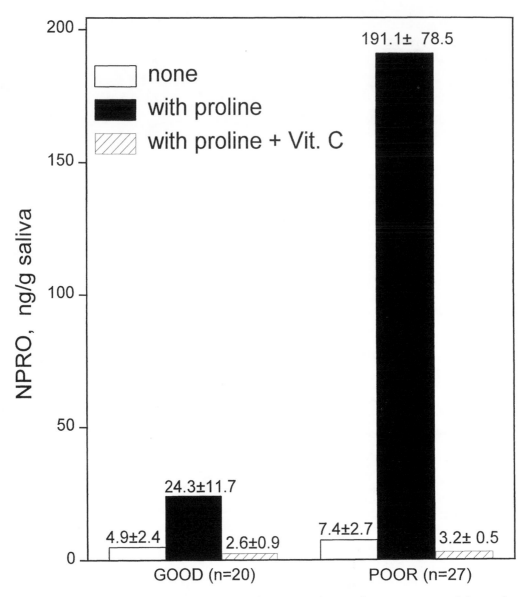

FIGURE 3. Effect of oral hygiene on nitrosamine formation in the mouth. (Adapted from Nair, J., Havovi, S., Chakradeo, P., Jakhi, S. A., and Bhide, S. V., in *Nitroso Compounds: Biological Mechanisms, Exposure and Cancer Etiology*, O'Neill, I. K. and Bartsch, H., Eds., International Agency for Research on Cancer, Lyon, 1992, 11.)

V. ON THE CONTROVERSY OF WHETHER NICOTINE IS NITROSATED IN HUMANS *IN VIVO*

Nicotine, which has a tertiary amino group, contributes 85 to 95% of the alkaloid content in the tobacco species *N. tabaccum*.[6]

N. rustica, which is frequently used for chewing in India and as snuff in Sudan, has higher levels of nicotine.[33] Nicotine has been shown to react with nitrite at acidic pH to yield NNN and NNK,[34] and therefore endogenous formation of these TSNA has been hypothesized.[6,9,35] 4-(*N*-methylnitrosamino)-4-(3-

pyridyl)butyric acid (Iso-NNAC) could be formed from nicotine via its nitrosated product 4-(N- methyl-nitrosamino)-4-(3-pyridyl)-1-butanol or via nitrosation of its major metabolite, cotinine.[36] Using urinary excretion of Iso-NNAC as a probe, it has not been demonstrated that in subjects who refrained from smoking but received nicotine in gelatin capsules, endogenous nitrosation did take place.[37] However, in the same study 44 to 163 ng of Iso-NNAC was found in four out of 20 urine samples of cigarette smokers (18 to 21 cigarettes per day), and was attributed to the inhalation of preformed Iso-NNAC absorbed from cigarette smoke. The mean concentration of Iso-NNAC reported in mainstream smoke by the authors was 2.2 ng per cigarette. In an earlier study, the level of Iso-NNAC was reported to be <1 ng per cigarette[36] (U.S. blend tobacco) and 3 ng per cigarette (French black tobacco). Thus, the relatively high amounts of Iso-NNAC detected in some urine samples do not fit the authors' postulate that these levels are uniquely derived from preformed Iso-NNAC in tobacco smoke.[37] Furthermore, the absence of Iso-NNAC in subjects who received nicotine only must be cautiously interpreted, as the two factors in tobacco smoke that enhance nitrosation, NO_x and thiocyanate, were absent when nicotine was administered.

Studies by Jacob et al.[38] recently demonstrated the occurrence of the minor tobacco alkaloids nornicotine, anatabine, and anabasine in the urine of cigarette smokers, tobacco chewers, and snuff dippers (Table 1). This is the first unequivocal demonstration that these easily nitrosatable alkaloids with a secondary amino group are either absorbed from tobacco or metabolically formed from the corresponding tertiary amines in the human body when tobacco is used, and hence will be available for nitrosation in the presence of nitrosating agents. When nicotine was given by i.v. infusion to volunteers, less than 1% of the alkaloid was converted into nornicotine via oxidative demethylation.[39] The twofold increased NPRO excretion in smokers (see Section II) may be an underestimate of the actual amounts of these secondary amines that could undergo endogenous nitrosation. As pKa values are inversely correlated with the rate of nitrosation of secondary amines, nornicotine with a pKa of 9.2 will nitrosate much more rapidly than proline (pKa 10.6).

VI. FORMATION OF NO BY INFLAMMATORY PROCESSES: THE NEED FOR REEVALUATING ENDOGENOUS NITROSATION

NO, which is overproduced via the inducible form of nitric oxide synthase during inflammatory processes that accompany in-

TABLE 1
Excretion of Tobacco Alkaloids Carrying a Nitrosatable Secondary Amino Group in Human Urine (μg/24 h) After the Use of Tobacco *Ad Libitum* by Healthy Volunteers

Alkaloids	Cigarette smokers (n = 22)	Tobacco chewers (n = 8)	Snuff dippers (n = 6)
Nornicotine	146 ± 99	388 ± 238	331 ± 175
Anabasine	7.3 ± 6.5	35 ± 41	22 ± 11
Anatabine	18 ± 16	109 ± 66	56 ± 20

Note: Data were extracted from Reference 38. Analysis was done by gas chromatography/mass spectrometry. Means ± SD are given.

fections by bacteria, parasites, or viruses, can increase the endogenous formation of nitrosamines.[12] Studies in infected animal models[40–42] and in humans[43–45] have shown that chronic infectious conditions yielded a higher amount of nitrosamines derived from nitrosating species (from NO) and nitrosatable amines. Most of the studies undertaken so far that demonstrated an increased endogenous nitrosation in tobacco users were carried out in healthy volunteers. No systematic studies have investigated the burden from endogenously formed nitrosamines in tobacco chewers and smokers who suffered from chronic infections. The observed increased excretion of nitroso compounds in these subjects who suffered from such conditions underscore the need for reevaluating the endogenous nitrosation potential in tobacco users.

VII. ENDOGENOUS FORMATION OF REACTIVE OXYGEN SPECIES IN CHEWERS OF BETEL QUID

Two major ingredients of BQ, areca nut and catechu, have been shown to produce superoxide anion (O_2^-) and H_2O_2 at alkaline pH *in vitro* that were detected by a chemiluminescence assay.[13] ROS, which may cause direct DNA damage in the oral mucosa and promote initiated oral epithelial cells,[46] appear to be a major source of DNA damage in chewers of BQ free of tobacco in Papua, New Guinea.[47] The large quantities of slaked lime used while chewing lead to a (temporary) oral pH of >9.5.[47] Strongly positive correlations were observed between pH, calcium hydroxide content of the lime samples, and the formation of O_2^-, H_2O_2, and 8OH-dG from BQ ingredients *in vitro*.[48] These results show the importance of pH for the ROS formation likely to occur via autoxidation, redox cycling, and iron-catalyzed Haber-Weiss and Fenton reactions (Figure 4). More recently, using the formation of ortho- and meta-tyrosines from phenylalanine (that was added to BQ while chewing), it has been demonstrated that OH radicals are formed in the oral cavity during the chewing of BQ.[49]

The frequency of micronuclei in exfoliated buccal mucosa cells was shown to be highest in chewers of BQ plus lime, followed by chewers of tobacco, suggesting a role of ROS in oxidative DNA and chromosomal damage.[47,50] A study by Thomas and MacLennan[47] further supports the role of ROS generated while chewing BQ in oral cancer. They found that in BQ chewers of Papua, New Guinea, tumors arose more frequently in the location of the mouth where lime is applied while chewing.

Epidemiological studies suggested that tobacco and other BQ ingredients could act synergistically in the causation of oral cancer.[1] It is possible that nitrosamines in tobacco (TSNA) and ROS generated from BQ ingredients during chewing concomitantly cause DNA damage to oral epithelial cells that leads to malignant growth. Indeed, the induction of tumors in the hamster cheek pouch by simultaneous application of H_2O_2 and NNK has been reported,[51] and the chemical activation of NNN by H_2O_2 via the Fenton reaction was shown to occur *in vitro*.[52] Also, DNA strand breaks in human lung fibroblast cells treated with NNN or NNK in combination with a ROS-generating system (xanthine/xanthine oxidase) were enhanced.[53]

VIII. CONCLUSIONS AND PERSPECTIVES

Experimental studies and investigations in healthy volunteers provided evidence that smoking and the chewing of tobacco enhance nitrosation reactions and lead to an increased burden of carcinogenic nitrosamines. The inability to demonstrate an *in vivo* nitrosation of nicotine should not be taken as finite evidence that the formation of nitrosamines does not occur in tobacco us-

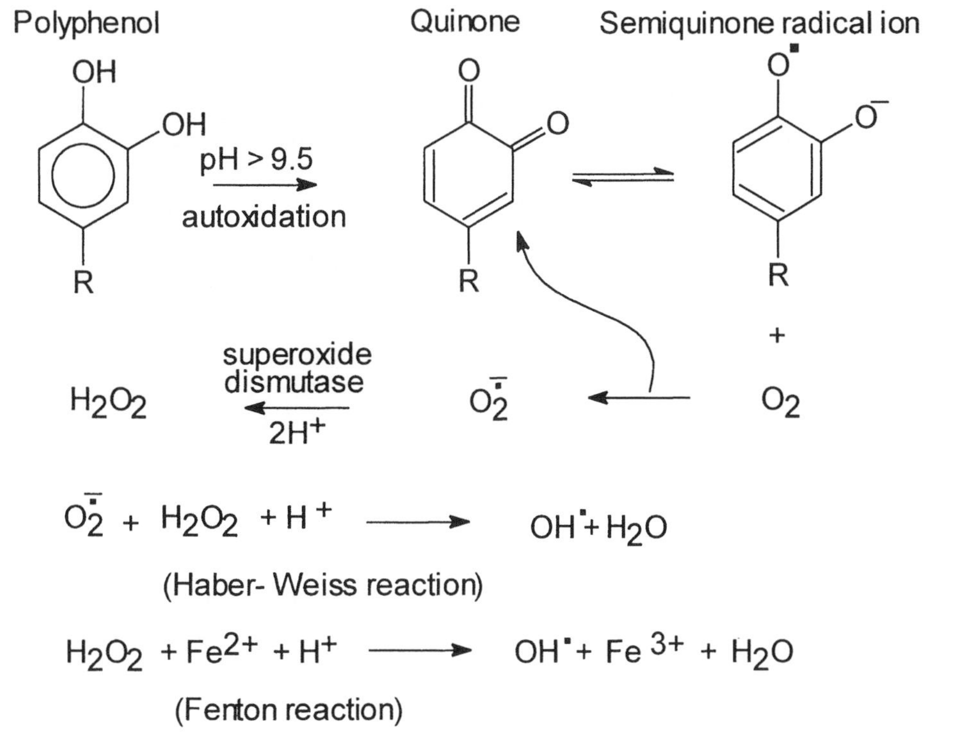

FIGURE 4. Scheme for the formation of reactive oxygen species from polyphenols present in the BQ ingredients areca nut and Catechu.

ers, in view of the abundance of secondary amines in tobacco and tobacco smoke and the demonstrated absorption of the TSNA precursors nornicotine, anatabine, and anbasine in tobacco users. To resolve these problems, new biomarkers for discriminating between exposure to preformed and endogenously formed nitrosamines are required.

A third of all human cancers are caused by tobacco, and cessation of tobacco use is the only safe way of preventing tobacco-induced cancers. Despite this knowledge and all the attempted preventive measures, tobacco smoking is not declining worldwide. Possibly as a consequence of the prohibition of smoking in public places, the use of oral snuff is increasing in the U.S.[54] In 1988, the World Health Organization proposed implementation of an analysis of smokeless tobacco products and the regulation of harmful

substances under government control.[55] Such regulatory measures would appear beneficial if applied to the known preformed carcinogens in tobacco. However, the uncertainty of the extent to which endogenously formed nitroso compounds and ROS contribute to the tobacco-associated cancer risk complicates the development of less harmful tobacco products.

ACKNOWLEDGMENTS

Most of the work referred to by J. Nair and U. J. Nair was carried out during tenures of fellowships at the International Agency for Research on Cancer (IARC) in Lyon, France. The authors wish to acknowledge the collaborative support provided by Dr. S. V. Bhide, Bombay, India, and the colleagues of the ex-Unit of Environmental Carcinogens and Host Factors at IARC.

REFERENCES

1. **International Agency for Research on Cancer,** *Tobacco Habits Other Than Smoking: Betel Quid and Areca Nut Chewing and Some Related Nitrosamines,* IARC Monograph, Lyon, 1985, 37.

2. **International Agency for Research on Cancer,** *Tobacco Smoking,* IARC Monograph, Lyon, 1986, 38.

3. **Doll, R. and Peto, R.,** The cause of cancer: quantitative estimates of avoidable risks of cancer in United States today, *JNCI,* 66, 1191, 1982.

4. **Wynder, E. L. and Gori, G. B.,** Contribution of the environment to cancer: an epidemiological exercise, *JNCI,* 58, 825, 1977.

5. **Hoffmann, D. and Wynder, E. L.,** Chemical constituents and bioactivity of tobacco smoke, in *Tobacco, A Major International Health Hazard,* Zaridze, D. and Peto. R., Eds., International Agency for Research on Cancer, Lyon, 1986, 145.

6. **Hoffmann, D., Brunnemann, K. D., Prokopczyk, B., and Djordjevic, M.V.,** Tobacco specific *N*-nitrosamines and areca-derived *N*-nitrosamines: chemistry, biochemistry, carcinogenicity, and relevance to humans, *J. Toxicol. Environ. Health,* 45, 1, 1994.

7. **Brunnemann, K. D., Prokopczyk, B., Hoffmann, D., Nair, J., Ohshima, H., and Bartsch, H.,** Laboratory studies on oral cancer and smokeless tobacco, in *Mechanisms in Tobacco Carcinogenesis,* Hoffmann, D. and Harris, C. C., Eds., Banbury Report 23, 1986, 197.

8. **Idris, I. M., Nair, J., Ohshima, H., Friesen, M., Brouet, I., Faustman, E. M., and Bartsch, H.,** Unusually high levels of carcinogenic tobacco-specific nitrosamines in Sudan snuff (toombak), *Carcinogenesis,* 12, 1115, 1991.

9. **Hecht, S. S. and Hoffmann, D.,** Tobacco-specific nitrosamines, an important group of carcinogens in tobacco and tobacco smoke, *Carcinogenesis,* 9, 875, 1988.

10. **Hoffmann, D. and Hecht, S. S.,** Advances in tobacco carcinogenesis, in *Handbook of Experimental Pharmacology,* Springer-Verlag, New York, 94, 63, 1990.

11. **Preston-Martin, S.,** Evaluation of the evidence that tobacco-specific nitrosamines (TSNA) cause cancer in humans, *CRC Crit. Rev. Toxicol.,* 21, 295, 1991.

12. **Ohshima, H. and Bartsch, H.,** Chronic infections and inflammatory process as cancer risk factors: possible role of nitric oxide in carcinogenesis, *Mutat. Res.,* 305, 253, 1994.

13. **Nair, U. J., Floyd, R. A., Nair, J., Bussachini, V., Friesen, M., and Bartsch, H.,** Formation of reactive oxygen species and of 8-hydroxydeoxyguanosine in DNA *in vitro* with betel quid ingredients, *Chem. Biol. Interact.,* 63, 157, 1987.

14. **Cadet, J.,** DNA damage caused by oxidation, deamination, ultraviolet radiation and photo exited psoralens, in *DNA Adducts, Identification and Biological Significance,* Hemminki, K., Dipple, A., Shuker, D. E. G., Kadlubar, F. F., Segerback, D., and Bartsch, H., Eds., IARC Sci. Publ., 125, International Agency for Research on Cancer, Lyon, 1994, 245.

15. **Ohshima, H. and Bartsch, H.,** Quantitative estimation of endogenous nitrosation in humans by monitoring *N*-nitrosoproline excreted in the urine, *Cancer Res.,* 41, 3658, 1981.

16. **Hoffmann, D. and Brunnemann, K. D.,** Endogenous formation of *N*-nitrosoproline in cigarette smokers, *Cancer Res.,* 43, 5570, 1983.

17. **Ladd, K. F., Newmark, H. L., and Archer, M. C.,** *N*-Nitrosation of proline in smokers and non smokers, *JNCI,* 73, 83, 1984.

18. **Bartsch, H., Ohshima, H., Munoz, N., Crespi, M., Cassale, V., Ramazzotti,V., Lambert, R., Minaire, Y., Forichon, J., and Walters, C. L.,** *In vivo* nitrosation, precancerous lesions and cancers of gastrointestinal tract: ongoing studies and preliminary results, in *N-Nitroso Compounds, Occurrence, Biological Effects, and Relevance to Human Cancers,* O'Neill, I. K., von Borstel, R. C., Miller, C. T., Long, L. E., and Bartsch, H., IARC Sci. Publ. 57, International Agency for Research on Cancer, Lyon, 1984, 955.

19. **Nair, J., Ohshima, H., Pignatelli, B., Friesen, M., Malaveille, C., Calmels, S.,**

and **Bartsch, H.,** Modifiers of endogenous carcinogen formation: studies on *in vivo* nitrosation in tobacco users, in *Mechanisms in Tobacco Carcinogenesis,* Hoffmann, D. and Harris, C. C ., Eds., Banbury Report 23, 1986, 45.

20. **Tsuda, M. and Kurashima, Y.,** Tobacco smoking, chewing and snuff dipping: factors contributing to the endogenous formation of *N*-nitroso compounds, *Crit. Rev. Toxicol.,* 21, 243, 1991.

21. **Hecht, S. S., Ornaf, R. M., and Hoffmann, D.,** Chemical studies on tobacco smoke. XXXIII. *N'*-nitrosonornicotine in tobacco: analysis of possible contributing factors and biological implications, *JNCI,* 54, 1237, 1974.

22. **Tricker, A. R., Haubner, R., Spiegelhalder, B., and Preussmann, R.,** The occurrence of tobacco-specific nitrosamines in oral tobacco products and their potential formation under simulated gastric conditions, *Food Chem. Toxicol.,* 26, 861, 1988.

23. **Nair, J., Ohshima, H., Friesen, M., Croisy, A., Bhide, S. V., and Bartsch, H.,** Tobacco-specific and betel-nut specific *N*-nitroso compounds: occurrence in saliva and urine of betel quid chewers and formation *in vitro* by nitrosation of betel quid, *Carcinogenesis,* 6, 295, 1985.

24. **Nair, J., Nair, U. J., Ohshima, H., Bhide, S. V., and Bartsch, H.,** Endogenous nitrosation in the oral cavity of chewers while chewing betel quid with or without tobacco, in *The Relevance of* N-*Nitroso Compounds in Human Cancer: Exposure and Mechanisms,* Bartsch, H., O'Neill, I. K., and Schulte-Hermann, R., Eds., IARC Sci. Publ. 84, International Agency for Research on Cancer, Lyon, 1987, 465.

25. **Prokopczyk, B., Rivenson, A., Bertinato, P., Brunnemann, K. D., and Hoffmann, D.,** 3-(Methylnitrosamino)propionitrile: occurrence in saliva of betel quid chewers, carcinogenicity and DNA methylation, *Cancer Res.,* 47, 467, 1987.

26. **Stich, H. F., Parida, B. B., and Brunnemann, K. D.,** Localized formation of micronuclei in oral mucosa and tobacco specific nitrosamines in saliva of "reverse" smokers, khaini tobacco chewers and gudakhu users, *Int. J. Cancer,* 50, 172, 1992.

27. **Osterdahl, B.-G. and Slorach, S.,** Tobacco specific *N*-nitrosamines in the saliva of habitual male snuff dippers, *Food Add. Contam.,* 5, 581, 1988.

28. **Carmella, S. G., Kagan, S. S., Kagan, M., Foiles, P. G., Palladino, G., Quart, A. M., Quart, E., and Hecht, S. S.,** Mass spectrometric analysis of tobacco-specific nitrosamine haemoglobin adducts in snuff dippers, smokers and non-smokers, *Cancer Res.,* 50, 5438, 1990.

29. **Nair, J., Havovi, S., Chakradeo, P., Jakhi, S. A., and Bhide, S. V.,** Increased endogenous formation of *N*-nitroso compounds in the oral cavity of subjects with poor oral hygiene, in *Nitroso Compounds: Biological Mechanisms, Exposure and Cancer Etiology,* O'Neill, I. K. and Bartsch, H., Eds., IARC Tech. Rep. 11, International Agency for Research on Cancer, Lyon, 1992, 11.

30. **Calmels, S., Ohshima, H., Vincent, P., Gounot, A.-M., and Bartsch, H.,** Screening of microorganisms for nitrosation catalysis at pH 7 and kinetic studies on nitrosamine formation from secondary amines by *E. coli* strains, *Carcinogenesis,* 6, 911, 1985.

31. **Calmels, S., Ohshima, H., Crespi, M., Leclerc, H., Cattoen, C., and Bartsch, H.,** Nitrosamine formation by microorganisms isolated from human gastric juice and urine: biochemical studies on the bacteria catalysed nitrosation, in *The Relevance of* N-*Nitroso Compounds in Human Cancer: Exposure and Mechanisms,* Bartsch, H. O'Neill, I. K. and Schulte-Hermann R., Eds., IARC Sci. Publ. 84, International Agency for Research on Cancer, Lyon, 1987, 391.

32. **Calmels, S., Ohshima, H., Henry, Y., and Bartsch, H.,** Characterization of bacterial cytochrome CD_1-nitrate reductase as one enzyme responsible for catalysis of nitrosation of secondary amines, *Carcinogenesis,* 17, in press, 1996.

33. **Sisson, V. A. and Seversson, R. F.,** Alkaloid composition of Nicotiana species, *Beitr. Tabakforsch.,* 14, 327, 1990.

34. **Hecht, S. S. ,Chen, C. B., Ornaf, R. M., Jacobs, E., Adams, J. D., and Hoffmann, D.,** Reaction of nicotine and sodium nitrite: formation of nitrosamines and fragmentation of pyrrolidine ring, *J. Org. Chem.*, 43, 72, 1978.

35. **Djordjevic, M. V., Brunnemann, K. D., and Hoffmann, D.,** Identification and analysis of a nicotine derived *N*-nitrosamino acid and other nitrosamino acids in tobacco, *Carcinogenesis*, 10, 1725, 1989.

36. **Djordjevic, M. V., Sigountos, C. W., Brunnemann, K. D., and Hoffmann, D.,** Formation of 4-(methylnitrosamino)-4-(3-pyridyl) butyric acid *in vitro* and in main stream cigarette smoke, *J. Agric. Food. Chem.*, 39, 209, 1991.

37. **Tricker, A. R., Scherer, G., Conze, C., Adlkofer, F., Pachinger, A., and Klus, H.,** Evaluation of 4-(methylnitrosamino)-4-(3-pyridyl) butyric acid as a potential monitor of endogenous nitrosation of nicotine and its metabolites, *Carcinogenesis*, 14, 1409, 1993.

38. **Jacob, P., III, Yu, L., Liang, G., Shulgin, A. T., and Benowitz, N. L.,** Gas chromatographic-mass spectrometric method for determination of anabasine, anatabine and other tobacco alkaloids in urine of smokers and smokeless tobacco users, *J. Chromatogr.*, 619, 49, 1993.

39. **Neurath, G. B., Orth, D., and Pein, F. G.,** Detection of nornicotine in human urine after infusion of nicotine, in *Effects of Nicotine and Biological Systems*, Adlkofer, F. and Thurau, K., Eds., Birkhäuser, Basel, 1991, 45.

40. **Wu, Y., Brouet, I., Calmels, S., Bartsch, H., and Ohshima, H.,** Increased endogenous *N*-nitrosamine and nitrate formation by induction of nitric oxide synthase in rats with acute hepatic injury caused by *Propionibacterium acnes* and lipopolysaccharide administration, *Carcinogenesis*, 14, 7, 1993.

41. **Leaf, C., Wishnok, J. S., and Tannenbaum, S. R.,** Endogenous incorporation of nitric oxide from L-arginine into *N*-nitrosomorpholine stimulated by *Escherichia coli* lipopolysaccharide in the rat, *Carcinogenesis*, 12, 537, 1991.

42. **Liu, R. H., Baldwin, B., Tennant, B. C., and Hotchkiss, J. H.,** Elevated formation of nitrate and nitrosodimethylamine in woodchucks (*Marmota monax*) associated with chronic woodchuck hepatitis virus infection, *Cancer Res.*, 51, 3925, 1991.

43. **Ohshima, H., Calmels, S., Pignatelli, B., Vincent, P., and Bartsch, H.,** *N*-Nitrosamine formation in urinary tract infections, in *The Relevance of* N-*Nitroso Compounds in Human Cancer: Exposure and Mechanisms*, Bartsch, H., O'Neill, I. K. and Schulte-Hermann, R., Eds., IARC Sci. Publ. 84, International Agency for Research on Cancer, Lyon, 1987, 384.

44. **Tricker, A. R., Mostafa, M. H., Spiegelhalder, B., and Preussmann, R.,** Urinary excretion of nitrate, nitrite and *N*-nitroso compounds in schistosomiasis and bilharzia bladder cancer patients, *Carcinogenesis*, 10, 547, 1989.

45. **Srivatanukul, P., Ohshima, H., Khlat, M., Parkin, M., Sukaryodhin, S., Brouet, I., and Bartsch, H.,** *Opisthorchis viverrini* infestation and endogenous nitrosamine as risk factors for cholangiocarcinoma in Thailand, *Int. J. Cancer*, 48, 821, 1991.

46. **Stich, H. F. and Anders, F.,** The involvement of reactive oxygen species in oral cancer of betel quid/tobacco chewers, *Mutat. Res.*, 214, 47, 1989.

47. **Thomas, S. J. and MacLennan, R.,** Slaked lime and betel nut cancer in Papua New Guinea, *Lancet*, 340, 577, 1992.

48. **Nair, U. J., Friesen, M., Richard, I., MacLennan, R., Thomas, S., and Bartsch, H.,** Effect of lime composition on the formation of reactive oxygen species from areca nut extract *in vitro*, *Carcinogenesis*, 11, 2145, 1990.

49. **Nair, U. J., Nair, J., Friesen, M. D., Bartsch, H., and Ohshima, H.,** Ortho- and meta-tyrosine formation from phenyl alanine in human saliva as a marker of hydroxy radical generation during betel quid chewing, *Carcinogenesis*, 16, 1195, 1995.

50. **Nair, U., Obe, G., Nair, J., Maru, G. B., Bhide, S. V., Pieper, R., and Bartsch, H.,** Evaluation of frequency of micronucleated

oral mucosa cells as a marker for genotoxic damage in chewers of betel quid with or without tobacco, *Mutat. Res.*, 261, 163, 1991.

51. **Padma, P. R., Lalitha, V. S., Amonkar, A. J., and Bhide, S. V.,** Carcinogenic studies on the two tobacco specific nitrosamines, *N′*-nitrosonornicotine and 4-(methylnitrosamino)-1-(3-pyridyl)-1-butanone, *Carcinogenesis*, 10, 1997, 1989.

52. **Nair, J., Nair, U. J., Amonkar, A. J., and Bhide, S. V.,** Activation of *N′*-nitrosonornicotine by hydrogen peroxide *in vitro*, in *Relevance to Human Cancer of N-Nitroso Compounds, Tobacco Smoke and Mycotox-ins*, O'Neill, I. K., Chen, J., and Bartsch, H., Eds., IARC Sci. Publ. 105, International Agency for Research on Cancer, Lyon, 1991, 516.

53. **Weitberg, A. B. and Corvese, D.,** Oxygen radicals potentiate the genetic toxicity of tobacco-specific nitrosamines, *Clin. Genet.*, 43, 88, 1993.

54. **Marwick, C.,** Increasing use of chewing tobacco, especially among younger persons, alarms surgeon general, *JAMA*, 195, 1993.

55. **World Health Organization,** *Smokeless Tobacco Control*, WHO Tech. Rep. Ser. 773, 1988, 81.

RECENT STUDIES ON MECHANISMS OF BIOACTIVATION AND DETOXIFICATION OF 4-(METHYLNITROSAMINO)-1-(3-PYRIDYL)-BUTANONE (NNK), A TOBACCO-SPECIFIC LUNG CARCINOGEN

Critical Reviews in Toxicology, 26(2):163–181 (1996)

Recent Studies on Mechanisms of Bioactivation and Detoxification of 4-(Methylnitrosamino)-1-(3-Pyridyl)-1-Butanone (NNK), A Tobacco-Specific Lung Carcinogen

Stephen S. Hecht

American Health Foundation, Valhalla, NY 10595

ABSTRACT: This article reviews recent advances in the biochemistry and molecular biology of 4-(methylnitrosamino)-1-(3-pyridyl)-1-butanone (NNK), a tobacco-specific pulmonary carcinogen believed to be involved in the induction of lung cancer in smokers. Several aspects of NNK bioactivation are addressed, including identification of its metabolites in laboratory animals and humans, cytochrome P450 enzyme involvement in its metabolic activation, DNA and protein adduct formation, biological significance of the major DNA adducts formed, and mutations in oncogenes from tumors induced by NNK. Collectively, the presently available data provide a reasonably clear picture of NNK bioactivation in rodents, although there are still important gaps in our mechanistic understanding of NNK-induced tumorigenesis. The studies in rodents and primates have facilitated development of methods to assess NNK bioactivation in humans, which will be applicable to studies of lung cancer susceptibility and prevention.

KEY WORDS: 4-(Methylnitrosamino)-1-(3-pyridyl)-1-butanone, lung carcinogenesis, cytochromes P450, metabolic activation, glucuronidation, DNA adducts, hemoglobin adducts, K-*ras* oncogenes, O^6-methylguanine, DNA pyridyloxobutylation, DNA methylation.

I. INTRODUCTION

This review focuses on recent advances in the biochemistry and molecular biology of the tobacco-specific lung carcinogen 4-(methylnitrosamino)-1-(3-pyridyl)-1-butanone (NNK). Over 100 papers relevant to this topic have appeared in the past 5 years, attesting to a significant level of interest in the mechanisms by which NNK induces cancer. NNK is an important model compound for examining the mechanisms of pulmonary carcinogenesis in laboratory animals. It is also likely to play a significant role as a lung carcinogen in smokers.[1-3] Selected aspects of NNK biotransformation, adduct formation, and involvement in oncogene activation are discussed.

Abbreviations: NNK, 4-(methylnitrosamino)-1-(3-pyridyl)-1-butanone; **NNAL,** 4-(methylnitrosamino)-1-(3-pyridyl)-1-butanol; **NNAL-Gluc,** [4-(methylnitrosamino)-1-(3-pyridyl)but-1-yl]-β-O-D-glucosiduronic acid; **7-mG,** 7-methylguanine; O^6**-mG,** O^6-methylguanine; O^4**-mT,** O^4-methylthymine; **HPB,** 4-hydroxy-1-(3-pyridyl)-1-butanone; **GC-MS,** gas chromatography–mass spectrometry; **NNN,** N'-nitrosonornicotine; **AMMN,** acetoxymethylmethylnitrosamine; **NNKOAc,** 4-(acetoxymethylnitrosamino)-1-(3-pyridyl)-1-butanone.

1040-8444/96/$.50

II. IDENTIFICATION OF NNK METABOLITES

A. Laboratory Animals

An overview of NNK biotransformation pathways is presented in Figure 1. Reduction of the NNK carbonyl group giving NNAL is a major metabolic reaction in most systems examined, both *in vitro* and *in vivo*.[4-9] Laboratory animals treated with NNK rapidly convert a significant portion of it to NNAL, which can be detected in blood minutes after injection. NNAL also is a potent pulmonary carcinogen and can be regarded as a transport form of NNK.[6,10] An important advance was the identification of NNAL-Gluc as a urinary metabolite of NNK in mice and rats.[11] The amount of the NNK dose excreted as NNAL-Gluc in the urine reached a maximum of 22% at relatively high NNK doses but was substantially lower at NNK doses closer to human exposure levels. Subsequent investigations of NNK metabolism in the patas monkey demonstrated the presence of two diastereomers of NNAL-Gluc in urine, in contrast to the rat and mouse, which had mainly one diastereomer.[9] These two NNAL-Gluc diastereomers accounted for approximately 15 to 20% of the NNK dose when the amount administered was similar to human exposure levels, suggesting the use of NNAL-Gluc as a dosimeter for human uptake of NNK. As described later, this approach has been successful and has provided some new insights into NNK metabolism in humans. NNAL-Gluc has also been established as a major metabolite of NNK excreted into bile.[12] When other pathways of NNK metabolism are inhibited, the levels of NNAL plus NNAL-Gluc in urine increase.

Major urinary metabolites of NNK in rodents and primates result from α-hydroxylation of NNK and NNAL (hydroxylation on the methylene and methyl carbons adjacent to the *N*-nitroso group), pyridine-*N*-oxidation of NNK and NNAL, and glucuronidation of NNAL (see Figure 1).[4,9,11,13] Unchanged NNK is rarely detected in urine. A minor urinary metabolite of NNK was recently identified as 6-hydroxyNNK, resulting from hydroxylation of the 6-position of the pyridine ring.[13] This is the only known pyridyl hydroxylated metabolite of NNK and, by analogy to studies on nicotine metabolism, may be formed by bacterial metabolism of NNK. Ongoing studies of NNK metabolism *in vitro* and *in vivo* in rodents and primates have failed to demonstrate significant amounts of metabolites resulting from hydroxylation β- or γ- to the *N*-nitroso group.

A surprising observation was made by Peterson et al. in a study of NNK metabolism by rat pancreatic microsomes, which were being investigated for their ability to metabolically activate NNK by α-hydroxylation.[14] Although this pathway could not be demonstrated, two new metabolites of NNK and one new metabolite of NNAL were observed. These were identified as $NADP^+$ or NADPH analogs, in which nicotinamide was replaced by either NNK or NNAL (see Figure 1). The formation of the $NADP^+$ analogs was catalyzed by NAD^+ glycohydrolase. Other pyridine compounds have been shown previously to be substrates for this reaction and its biological relevance is unclear. The NNK and NNAL $NADP^+$ analogs, which are also formed in rat liver microsomal incubations, elute from HPLC near some of the other NNK metabolites and can readily be mistaken for other metabolites if sufficient care is not taken in metabolite characterization.

A potentially important observation was the report by Murphy et al. of a glucuronide of α-hydroxymethylNNK, detected in hepatocytes and urine of phenobarbital pretreated rats dosed with NNK.[15] The isolation of this metabolite establishes conclusively that α-hydroxymethylNNK is a metabolite of NNK. This had been deduced previously from consideration of the chemistry of model compounds. More importantly, Murphy's

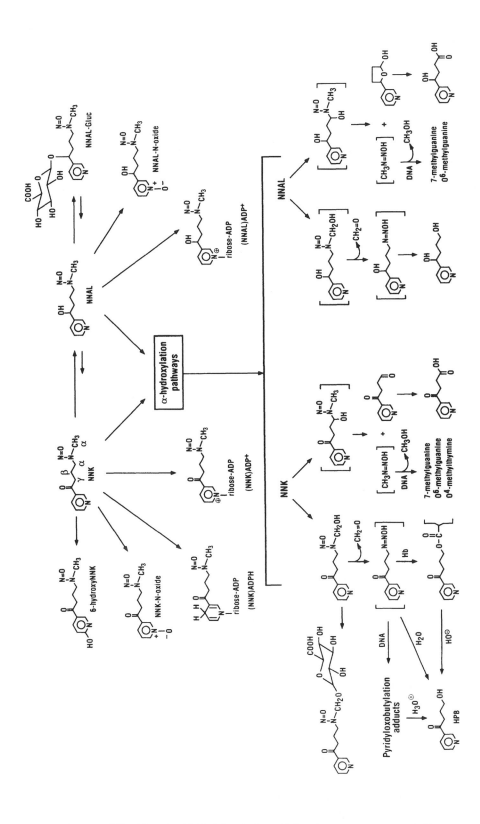

FIGURE 1. NNK metabolism pathways, as determined in rodents and primates. Compounds in brackets are postulated intermediates.

results show that α-hydroxymethylNNK has sufficient lifetime to be converted to a stable transport form, which could be involved in the carcinogenic activity of NNK. Previously, it had been assumed that α-hydroxylated metabolites of NNK would decompose and react with cellular macromolecules at the site of their formation. α-Hydroxyglucuronides of some other nitrosamines have been observed by Wiessler and co-workers.[16]

All published data are consistent with the hypothesis that α-hydroxylation is the major metabolic activation pathway of NNK. Intermediates and products involved in this bioactivation route are summarized in Figure 1. The enzymology of α-hydroxylation and its role in adduct formation by NNK are discussed herein.

B. Humans

Based on the detection of substantial amounts of NNAL-Gluc diastereomers in patas monkey urine after treatment with low doses of NNK, methodology was developed to investigate the presence of NNAL-Gluc in human urine.[17,18] This led to the detection of both NNAL-Gluc and NNAL in the urine of smokers, but not in nonsmokers who have not been exposed passively to tobacco smoke. NNAL and NNAL-Gluc have been detected in the urine of all of the over 100 smokers analyzed to date. In one study, amounts of NNAL-Gluc ranged from 0.16 to 19.0 pmol/mg creatinine (mean ± S.D., 2.81 ± 2.92), whereas NNAL levels varied from 0.08 to 4.89 pmol/mg creatinine (mean ± S.D., 0.95 ± 1.15).[18] These levels are consistent with the amounts of NNK reported in mainstream cigarette smoke and support the proposal that uptake of NNK by a smoker results in a lifetime dose similar to that which can induce lung tumors in laboratory animals. Levels of NNAL plus NNAL-Gluc in urine are correlated with cotinine in urine.

The ratio of NNAL-Gluc to NNAL could be an indicator of detoxification potential for NNK, since NNAL-Gluc is expected to be less carcinogenic than either NNK or NNAL (although this has not been tested to date). NNAL-Gluc/NNAL ratios appear to segregate into two phenotypes, as illustrated in Figure 2.[18] Presumably, smokers in the higher ratio group would be protected to some extent from the carcinogenic effects of NNK and NNAL. The ratio phenotype is now being applied as a biomarker in molecular epidemiology studies.

NNAL and NNAL-Gluc have been identified in the urine of nonsmokers exposed to environmental tobacco smoke in a study that roughly duplicated conditions in a heavily smoke-polluted room.[19] This study established the presence of a lung carcinogen — NNAL — in the urine of nonsmokers exposed to environmental tobacco smoke, demonstrating that nonsmokers take up and metabolize NNK. The results provided experimental support for the proposal that environmental tobacco smoke can cause lung cancer. In another investigation, NNAL and NNAL-Gluc levels were quantified in the urine of people from Sudan who used an oral tobacco product — toombak — known to contain unusually high levels of NNK.[20] The NNAL and NNAL-Gluc levels in urine demonstrated that carcinogen uptake by this group was among the largest ever observed, far exceeding uptake of aflatoxin, as one example. Further analysis of this urine demonstrated that both NNAL-Gluc diastereomers were present, as seen in the patas monkey.

III. ENZYME INVOLVEMENT IN NNK BIOACTIVATION

A. Laboratory Animals

Extensive studies have now clearly shown that α-hydroxylation of NNK is catalyzed mainly by cytochromes P450.[21-34] Py-

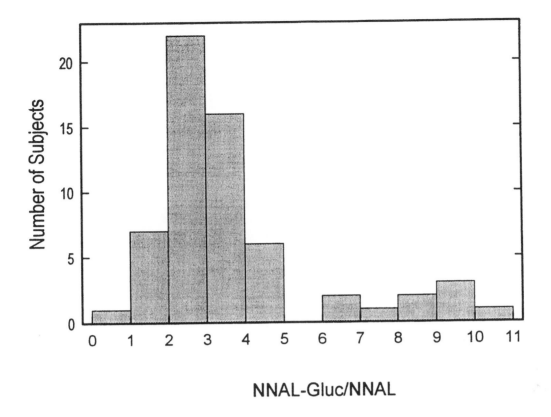

FIGURE 2. Distribution of NNAL-Gluc/NNAL ratios in the urine of 61 smokers. Each bar represents the number of subjects with ratios between 0-1, 1-2, etc.

ridine-*N*-oxidation is also mediated by cytochromes P450 in certain cases. These enzymes have generally not been implicated in the carbonyl reduction of NNK to NNAL. Studies on the role of cytochromes P450 in NNK metabolism are summarized in Table 1. Several points are noteworthy. In rat and mouse lung, catalysis of α-hydroxylation by CYP2B1 and CYP2A1, or immunochemically related forms, has been a consistent finding. CYP2B1 appears to be consistently involved mainly as a catalyst of methylene hydroxylation in the lung, whereas CYP2A1 has been implicated in both methylene and methyl hydroxylation. In liver, several forms including CYP1A2 play prominent roles. It is likely that some important cytochrome P450 activities involved in NNK bioactivation in the lung have not been characterized yet because the present evidence cannot fully account for the inhibition of NNK

metabolism in lung after treatment of rodents with inhibitors such as phenethyl isothiocyanate. Several cytochromes P450 appear to play no major role in NNK metabolism in rodents. These include CYP1A1, 2C11, and 2E1. The latter is involved in the metabolism of some other nitrosamines, such as *N*-nitrosodimethylamine.[35]

B. Humans

A number of studies have examined human cytochrome P450 involvement in NNK metabolism. These are summarized in Table 1. CYP1A2 has the highest catalytic activity for methyl hydroxylation. Other studies have consistently demonstrated activity for CYP2A6 and CYP2E1.

The role of CYP2D6 is of interest because some studies have shown that exten-

TABLE 1
Cytochrome P-450 Involvement in NNK Metabolism

Experimental System	Main P450 Involvement CYP-		No Involvement CYP-	Ref.
A. Rat				
Lung microsomes/antibody inhibition[a]	2B	Methylene hydroxylation	4B1	21
Lung microsomes/antibody inhibition[a]	1A2[b], 2A1, 2B1	Methylene hydroxylation	1A1, 2C11, 2E1, 3A	22
Liver microsomes/antibody inhibition[a]	2A1	Methyl hydroxylation		23
	1A2, 3A	Methylene hydroxylation	1A1, 2B1, 2C11, 2E1	
	1A2, 2A1, 3A	Methyl hydroxylation		
Reconstituted system using CYP2B1	2B1	Methylene hydroxylation, Methyl hydroxylation, Pyridine-N-oxidation		24
Ad293 cells transfected with CYP2B1 cDNA	2B1	Pyridine-N-oxidation		25
Nasal mucosa microsomes/antibody inhibition[a]	1A2, 2A1, 3A	Methylene hydroxylation	1A1, 2B1, 2C11, 2E1	22
	1A2	Methylene hydroxylation		
B. Mouse				
Lung microsomes/antibody inhibition[a]	2B1,2	α-Hydroxylation	1A2	26

168

System	P450	Reaction	Related forms	Ref.
Lung microsomes/antibody inhibition[a]	2B1 } 2A1 }	Methylene hydroxylation	1A1, 2C11, 2E1, 1A2, 3A	27
	2A1	Methyl hydroxylation		
		C. Rabbit		
Reconstituted system using nasal mucosa P450s	NMa	Methylene and methyl hydroxylation		28
	NMb	Methylene hydroxylation		
		D. Human		
B-Lymphoblastoid cell lines transfected with human cDNA	1A2 2A6 } 2D6 2E1 }	Metabolic activation		29
Hepatoma cells transfected with human cDNA	1A2> 2A6, 2B7, 2E1, 2F1 3A5 }	Methyl hydroxylation	2C8, 2C9, 2D6, 3A3, 3A4, 4B1	30
B-Lymphoblastoid cell lines transfected with human cDNA	2D6	Methylene hydroxylation Methyl hydroxylation		31
Liver microsomes/mutagenicity/antibody inhibition	2A6 2E1 1A2 }	Metabolic activation	2D6, 3A4, P450$_{MP}$	32
C3H/10T1/2 cells transfected with human CYP2A6	2A6	Metabolic activation		33
C3H/10T1/2 cells transfected with human CYP2A6	2A6	Metabolic activation		34

a Results pertain to specific P450s or immunochemically related forms.
b CYP1A2 has not been detected in rat lung.

sive metabolizers of debrisoquine are at higher risk for lung cancer. Debrisoquine metabolism is catalyzed by CYP2D6. Some controversy has arisen over the ability of CYP2D6 to catalyze NNK bioactivation. It now appears clear that CYP2D6 can metabolically activate NNK, but to a lesser extent than several other cytochromes P450.

It should be noted that NNK metabolism in human lung and liver microsomes is generally quantitatively different from that observed in rodents in that levels of carbonyl reduction to NNAL are usually greater whereas levels of α-hydroxylation are lower than in rodents. This may be an experimental artifact or result from genuine rodent-human differences. Most human lung samples obtained so far were from long-term smokers whose capacity to metabolize NNK may have been affected by years of smoking.

Although isolated cytochromes P450 can metabolically activate NNK, a prominent role of these enzymes as catalysts for NNK bioactivation in humans has not been confirmed. A recent study suggested that lipoxygenase or related enzymes may play a significant role.[36]

IV. DNA AND PROTEIN ADDUCT FORMATION

A. Laboratory Animals

As illustrated in Figure 1, metabolic activation of NNK by methylene hydroxylation or methyl hydroxylation results in methylation or pyridyloxobutylation of DNA. The presence of methyl and pyridyloxobutyl adducts in DNA of tissues from animals treated with NNK has been established conclusively.[37-41] Methyl adducts identified are 7-mG, O^6-mG, and O^4-mT. Pyridyloxobutyl adducts are quantified by measurement of HPB released by either acid or neutral thermal hydrolysis. HPB quantitation has been

accomplished by radiochromatography and GC-MS. The structures of the adducts that release HPB upon acid hydrolysis have not been determined, due mainly to their instability at the nucleoside level and under conventional analytical conditions. However, HPB-releasing adducts can have a long lifetime in DNA, persisting in rat lung and liver for up to 4 weeks after a single injection of NNK.[42]

Levels of methyl adducts and pyridyloxobutyl adducts have been compared in rat lung, liver, and nasal mucosa as well as in mouse lung. In rats, the ratio of 7-mG to HPB released varied from 7 to 25 (lung) and from 13 to 49 (liver), with increasing dose.[43] The relatively greater levels of HPB at lower doses are probably due to the presence of high-affinity cytochromes P450 for methyl hydroxylation. Levels of HPB released from rat lung and liver DNA were equal to or greater than those of O^6-mG. In the nasal mucosa of rats treated chronically with NNK, levels of O^6-mG were five to seven times greater than those of HPB released.[44] In A/J mice treated with NNK, O^6-mG levels were persistent in lung for up to 15 d, and levels were consistently greater than those of HPB released.[45] The two adducts were formed and removed at different rates, consistent with differing cytochrome P450-mediated catalysis of the two metabolic activation pathways, as illustrated in Table 1.

Single-strand breaks have been observed in the DNA of rat and hamster liver after treatment with NNK, as well as in hepatocytes incubated with NNK.[46,47] Aldehydes generated in NNK metabolism via the α-hydroxylation pathway are partially involved in this mode of DNA damage.[48] Oxidative damage, as quantified by 8-oxodeoxyguanosine, has been detected in the lungs of rats and mice treated with NNK.[49]

Collectively, the available data indicate that NNK generates a wide spectrum of DNA damage in target tissues of rats and mice. Types of damage include methylation, pyridyloxobutylation, oxidation, and strand breakage. Some of these lesions are persistent and can cause miscoding and are probably responsible for cancer induction by NNK.

HPB-releasing hemoglobin adducts have been characterized in rats and mice treated with NNK.[50,51] One adduct is an ester, probably with aspartate or glutamate, that is hydrolyzed under mild basic conditions to release HPB.[52] The ester adduct comprises 20 to 40% of the total binding to hemoglobin; the remainder does not release HPB upon mild base hydrolysis and has not been fully characterized, although it is known that cysteine adducts are not formed to a significant extent.[53] As in DNA, the released HPB can be quantified by radiochromatography or GC–MS. Levels of HPB-releasing adducts in hemoglobin correlate with levels in DNA, although the relationship is not linear.[43] Following metabolic activation of NNK in rat hepatocytes, the α-hydroxynitrosamine or its transport form can migrate out of the hepatocyte and into the red blood cell, where it reacts with hemoglobin.[54] Hemoglobin itself also can activate NNK by methylene hydroxylation, resulting in methylation of the protein, but not in the formation of HPB-releasing adducts.[54] The HPB-releasing adduct has proven to be a useful indicator of extents of metabolic activation of NNK in studies with laboratory animals.

B. Humans

Two studies have reported significant differences between smokers and non-smokers in levels of 7-mG. In one, mean levels of 7-mG were $6.9/10^7$ nucleotides in total white blood cells, 4.7 in granulocytes, and 23.6 in lymphocytes of smokers compared with values of 3.4, 2.8, and $13.5/10^7$ nucleotides in nonsmokers.[55] A second study analyzed 7-mG in bronchial DNA samples and found mean levels of 17.3 adducts per 10^7 nucleotides in smokers and 4.7 in nonsmokers.[56]

Levels of O^6-mG in placental DNA did not differ between smokers and non-smokers.[57]

HPB-releasing adducts in human lung and trachea were quantified by GC-MS.[58] Adducts were higher in smokers than in nonsmokers, with levels of HPB-releasing adducts ranging from 0.004 to 0.072 pmol/ μmol guanine. These adducts could be produced from NNN as well as NNK.

Although the presently available data indicate that NNK produces DNA adducts in human lung, additional studies are necessary to investigate the relationship of adduct levels to smoking patterns, individual metabolic characteristics, mutations, and cancer. This approach is hindered to some extent by the difficulty in obtaining lung DNA from humans.

The quantitation of hemoglobin adducts thus presents an attractive alternative because hemoglobin is readily available. A GC-MS method for quantifying HPB-releasing adducts from human hemoglobin has been standardized.[59,60] HPB-releasing adducts have been quantified in smokers, snuff-dippers, and nonsmokers. The earlier work has been reviewed.[61] In two recent studies, levels of HPB-releasing hemoglobin adducts were quantified in nasal snuff users from Germany and in Sudanese toombak users.[20,62] Both groups showed elevated levels of hemoglobin adducts, similar to the earlier finding of elevated adduct levels in snuff-dippers from the U.S. In smokers, HPB-releasing adducts are elevated above background in only a subset of individuals and appear to be generally lower than in snuff users. This may relate to patterns of enzyme induction or inhibition due to constituents of tobacco smoke, but this requires further investigation.

V. BIOLOGICAL SIGNIFICANCE OF DNA METHYLATION AND PYRIDYLOXOBUTYLATION

The well-established miscoding properties of O^6-mG and the availability of sensitive immunochemical and HPLC-fluorescence methods for its quantitation encouraged fairly extensive investigation of its role in tumor induction by NNK following its initial identification in DNA of NNK-treated rodents.[37] Studies on the potential role of HPB-releasing DNA adducts have lagged behind since the requisite radiochemical or GC-MS methodology was developed later. Presently, it appears that both methylation and pyridyloxobutylation of DNA play some role in tumor induction by NNK in rats and mice.

Belinsky and co-workers carried out extensive investigations of the role of O^6-mG in lung tumor induction by NNK in rats.[63] They discovered that the Clara cells of the rat lung have a high capacity to activate NNK, presumably via a high-affinity cytochrome P450 enzyme, resulting in formation of substantial amounts of O^6-mG compared to other cell types of the lung. As Clara cells appear to have relatively low levels of the O^6-mG-DNA methyltransferase repair enzyme,[64] the adducts accumulated and persisted. A dose-response study of NNK-induced lung tumorigenesis demonstrated that there was a linear correlation between lung tumor induction at various doses and levels of O^6-mG in the Clara cells of the rat lung.[63] These results strongly suggest that O^6-mG is important in lung tumor induction by NNK. However, the tumors appear to arise mainly from the alveolar type II cells. These cells also metabolically activate NNK, but the linear correlation with tumor induction seen for O^6-mG in Clara cells was lacking. This apparent contradiction has not been resolved. However, it should be noted that carcinogenicity studies of [methylene-D$_2$]NNK and [methyl-D$_3$]NNK did not show any difference vs. NNK lung carcinogenicity in rats.[65] If methylation alone were important, we would have expected lower carcinogenicity of [methylene-D$_2$]NNK than NNK. It is likely that both methylation and pyridyloxobutylation of DNA are important in lung tumorigenesis by NNK. Pyridyloxobutyl

DNA adducts are highly mutagenic in several bacterial and mammalian test systems, with activity sometimes exceeding that of methyl adducts.[66,67] Pyridyloxobutylating compounds that do not methylate, such as NNN and NNKOAc, are carcinogenic, although generally less so than are methylating agents. An interesting property of pyridyloxobutylated DNA is its ability to inhibit O^6-mG-DNA methyltransferase; in this way it can act as a cocarcinogen with a methylating carcinogen.[68]

Belinsky and co-workers proposed that a combination of O^6-mG adducts and toxicity was important in the induction of nasal tumors in rats by NNK.[69] We also investigated this question by carrying out comparative studies of [methylene-D$_2$]NNK, [methyl-D$_3$]NNK, and NNK with respect to DNA adduct formation in the olfactory and respiratory portions of the nasal mucosa.[44] Bioassays had shown that [methylene-D$_2$]NNK was a stronger nasal carcinogen than NNK in the rat, whereas the activity of [methyl-D$_3$]NNK was similar to that of NNK. In the rats treated with [methylene-D$_2$]NNK, levels of O^6-mG in DNA from both the olfactory and respiratory portions of the nasal mucosa were significantly lower and levels of HPB-releasing DNA adducts higher than in the rats treated with equivalent doses of the less carcinogenic compounds NNK or [methyl-D$_3$]NNK. HPB-releasing DNA adducts also were formed in the nasal mucosa of rats treated with the nasal carcinogen NNN, which cannot methylate DNA. These results strongly support the role of DNA pyridyloxobutylation in rat nasal carcinogenesis by NNK.

Liu et al. studied the formation and persistence of O^6-mG in the livers of rats or hamsters treated with NNK.[70] High doses of NNK induce liver tumors in rats but not in hamsters. They found that O^6-mG persisted in hamster liver, but not in rat liver, due to more effective depletion of O^6-mG-DNA methyltransferase in the former. These results do not support the role of O^6-mG in

172

liver tumor induction by NNK in rats and suggest that other factors are involved. An immunochemical investigation of O^6-mG localization in various tissues of rats, mice, and hamsters treated with NNK was carried out by Van Bentham et al., who also concluded that factors other than O^6-mG must be important in the induction of tumors by NNK.[71]

In contrast to the results discussed, a relatively consistent picture has emerged in studies of DNA alkylation by NNK and lung tumor induction in the A/J mouse. Comparative tumorigenicity studies of [methylene-D_2]NNK, [methyl-D_3]NNK, and NNK demonstrated that [methylene-D_2]NNK was clearly less active than the other two compounds; levels of O^6-mG induced by this compound also were lower than those of the other two compounds.[72] An extensive comparative study of DNA adduct and tumor formation by NNK, AMMN (a DNA methylating agent), and NNKOAc (a DNA pyridyloxobutylating agent) in A/J mice clearly demonstrated the importance of persistence of O^6-mG in lung tumor formation.[45] Other studies have demonstrated the presence of O^6-mG in the alveolar type II cells, believed to be the precursor cells for adenomas and adenocarcinomas induced by NNK in A/J mice.[73] Analysis of mutations in the K-*ras* gene isolated from these tumors has shown a high prevalence of G to A transitions in the second base of codon 12, consistent with the expected mutation induced by O^6-mG.[73]

Collectively, the presently available results favor an important role for O^6-mG in tumor induction by NNK in the A/J mouse; studies in rats uniformly indicate that other factors, including DNA pyridyloxobutylation, are critical. Oxidative damage to DNA and single-strand breaks also may be involved in tumor induction by NNK. Although this discussion has focused on DNA damage and its role in carcinogenesis, other factors are clearly involved. Lung tumor induction by NNK in the C3H mouse resulted in *ras*

activation, as in the A/J mouse, yet the tumors were smaller and less numerous than in the A/J mouse.[74] In the C57BL/6 mouse, another "resistant" strain, O^6-mG formation by NNK was similar to that observed in the A/J mouse, but K-*ras* activation and tumor formation were less prevalent.[75]

VI. MUTATIONS IN ONCOGENES FROM NNK-INDUCED TUMORS

Following the initial studies of Belinsky et al. on activation of the K-*ras* oncogene in lung tumors induced by NNK in A/J mice,[76] a number of other studies have appeared, as summarized in Table 2. All studies have found that, when the K-*ras* gene is activated in lung tumors induced by NNK, the main activating mutation is GGT → GAT in codon 12. Several points are of interest in Table 2. Whereas activated K-*ras* genes have been detected in lung tumors from A/J mice and Syrian golden hamsters, they have not been found in lung tumors induced by NNK in F-344 rats. This suggests that pathways independent of K-*ras* activation are important in lung tumor induction by NNK in rats.

The presence of a GGT → GAT mutation in activated K-*ras* genes is consistent with the hypothesis that it results from direct reaction of the NNK-derived methylating agent with the gene, resulting in O^6-mG, which causes the observed G to A transition mutation. The pyridyloxobutylating agent NNKOAc induced both G to A transitions and G to T transversions in lung tumors from A/J mice, in contrast to the methylating agent AMMN, which caused exclusively G to A transitions, similar to NNK. These data also support the prominent role of DNA methylation in A/J mouse lung tumor induction by NNK.

GGT → GAT mutations in codon 12 have also been observed in hyperplasias induced by NNK in A/J mouse lung, consistent with the proposal that O^6-mG causes them. Other aspects are not as clear. For example, tumors from mice treated with NNK

173

TABLE 2
Mutation Induction by NNK and Related Compounds in K-*ras* and p53 Genes from Lung Tumors

Compound	Species	K-*ras*	p53	Ref.
NNK	A/J mouse	GGT → GAT, codon 12 (15/20)[a] — hyperplasias		73, 76
		GGT → GAT, codon 12 (7/10) — adenocarcinoma		
NNK	A/J mouse	GGT → GAT, codon 12 (26/28)		77
AMMN	A/J mouse	GGT → GAT, codon 12 (18/18)		
NNKOAc	A/J mouse	GGT → GAT, codon 12 (8/21)		
		GGT → TGT, codon 12 (5/21)		
		GGT → GTT, codon 12 (4/21)		
NNK	A/J mouse	GGT → GAT, codon 12 (19/19)		78
		GGT → GAT, codon 12 (11/34) — promotion by butylated hydroxytoluene		
NNK	A/J mouse	GGT → GAT, codon 12 (11/11)	Not detected	Ronai et al. unpublished
NNK	C3H mouse	GGT → GAT, codon 12 (46/59)		74
NNK	B6C3F1 mouse	GGT → GAT, codon 12 (1/22)	Not detected	79
NNK	C57BL/6 mouse	CAA → CGA, codon 12 (1/22)	Not detected	75
NNK	Syrian golden hamster	GGT → GAT, codon 12 (21/35)	Not detected	80
NNK	F344 rat	Not detected		81

[a] Numbers in parentheses: number of tumors having mutation/number of tumors analyzed.

and butylated hydroxytoluene, which promotes lung tumor development, had a lower frequency of K-*ras* mutations than did those in mice treated with NNK alone. In C3H mice, K-*ras* activation was seen in all tumors analyzed, but the tumors were not as numerous or aggressive as those in A/J mice, indicating that other factors are involved. K-*ras* activation was infrequent in C57BL/6 mouse lung tumors induced by NNK.

No studies have identified mutations in the p53 tumor suppressor gene in lung tumors induced in rodents by NNK.

In humans, activated K-*ras* genes with mutations in codon 12 have been detected in 16% of lung tumors and in 24% of adenocarcinomas of the lung.[82] The frequency of mutations is GGT → TGT (58%), → GTT (16%), and → GAT (19%). If the A/J mouse or Syrian golden hamster were the perfect model for human lung cancer, one could conclude perhaps that most of the observed mutations were due to compounds other than NNK. In the A/J mouse model, the methylation pathway is very important, but its relative importance in humans is unclear at present. If pyridyloxobutylation is important in human lung tumor induction, one might expect a larger proportion of G to T transversion mutations, as seen with NNKOAc. These aspects require further study. Presently, it is premature to attempt to relate mutational data from lung tumors induced in humans by cigarette smoke to data obtained in laboratory animals with individual constituents of smoke.

VII. CONCLUSIONS

The lung carcinogenicity of NNK in rats was first reported in 1980 and the first metabolism study also appeared that year.[4,83] In the last 14 years, a large number of studies have resulted in a fairly clear picture of NNK bioactivation, detoxification, and tumor induction mechanisms. NNK is metabolically activated by cytochrome P450 enzymes in rodent tissues. Human cytochromes P450 also can activate NNK, but their quantitative role is still unclear. The metabolic activation of NNK, by α-hydroxylation results in methylation and pyridyloxobutylation of DNA. There are competing partial detoxification reactions, including pyridine-*N*-oxidation and glucuronidation of NNAL. The DNA methylation and pyridyloxobutylation pathways are crucial in tumor induction by NNK and, depending on the species and tissue involved, one or the other pathway or both may have important roles. The adducts formed in these reactions can activate the K-*ras* oncogene in mice and hamsters, but this has not been observed in rats.

The mechanism by which NNK selectively induces lung tumors in rodents is not crystal clear, but several aspects favor this result: (1) rodent lung contains cytochromes P450 that efficiently metabolically activate NNK by α-hydroxylation, resulting in DNA binding; (2) the DNA adducts formed, such as O^6-mG and HPB-releasing adducts, can be highly persistent in lung or in particular cell types due to depletion of critical repair enzymes; and (3) these methyl and pyridyloxobutyl DNA adducts are mutagenic, leading to permanent alterations in important genes.

In parallel with DNA adduct formation in the lung, NNK also pyridyloxobutylates hemoglobin. The resulting adducts can be used to estimate the extent of NNK bioactivation under a given set of conditions, and possibly to estimate risk for tumor development. The ratio of NNAL-Gluc to NNAL in urine, as well as the total amount of these metabolites excreted, can also indicate the extent to which NNK is metabolically activated. The hemoglobin adducts and urinary metabolites of NNK are measurable in smokers and such biomarkers may be useful in extending our understanding of mechanisms of lung tumor induction in humans.

ACKNOWLEDGMENTS

Our studies on bioactivation of NNK are supported by National Cancer Institute Grant CA-44377.

REFERENCES

1. **Hecht, S. S. and Hoffmann, D.,** Tobacco-specific nitrosamines, an important group of carcinogens in tobacco and tobacco smoke, *Carcinogenesis,* 9, 875, 1988.

2. **Hecht, S. S. and Hoffmann, D.,** The relevance of tobacco-specific nitrosamines to human cancer, *Cancer Surv.,* 8, 273, 1989.

3. **Hecht, S. S. and Hoffmann, D.,** 4-(Methylnitrosamino)-1-(3-pyridyl)-1-butanone, a nicotine-derived tobacco-specific nitrosamine, and cancer of the lung and pancreas in humans, in *Origins of Human Cancer: A Comprehensive Review,* Brugge, J., Curran, T., Harlow, E., and McCormick, F., Eds., Cold Spring Harbor Laboratory Press, Cold Spring Harbor, NY, 1991, 745.

4. **Hecht, S. S., Young, R., and Chen, C. B.,** Metabolism in the F344 rat of 4-(N-methyl-N-nitrosamino)-1-(3-pyridyl)-1-butanone, a tobacco specific carcinogen, *Cancer Res.,* 40, 4144, 1980.

5. **Castonguay, A., Tjälve, H., and Hecht, S. S.,** Tissue distribution of the tobacco-specific carcinogen 4-(methylnitrosamino)-1-(3-pyridyl)-1-butanone, and its metabolites in F344 rats, *Cancer Res.,* 43, 630, 1983.

6. **Castonguay, A., Lin, D., Stoner, G. D., Radok, P., Furuya, K., Hecht, S. S., Schut, H. A. J., and Klaunig, J. E.,** Comparative carcinogenicity in A/J mice and metabolism by cultured mouse peripheral lung of N'-nitrosonornicotine, 4-(methylnitrosamino)-1-(3-pyridyl)-1-butanone and their analogs, *Cancer Res.,* 43, 1223, 1983.

7. **Castonguay, A., Stoner, G. D., Schut, H. A. J., and Hecht, S. S.,** Metabolism of tobacco-specific N-nitrosamines by cultured human tissues, *Proc. Natl. Acad. Sci. U.S.A.,* 80, 6694, 1983.

8. **Adams, J. D., LaVoie, E. J., and Hoffmann, D.,** On the pharmacokinetics of tobacco-specific N-nitrosamines in Fischer rats, *Carcinogenesis,* 6, 509, 1985.

9. **Hecht, S. S., Trushin, N., Reid-Quinn, C. A., Burak, E. S., Jones, A. B., Southers, J. L., Gombar, C. T., Carmella, S. G., Anderson, L. M., and Rice, J. M.,** Metabolism of the tobacco-specific nitrosamine 4-(methylnitrosamino)-1-(3-pyridyl)-1-butanone in the Patas monkey: pharmacokinetics and characterization of glucuronide metabolites, *Carcinogenesis,* 14, 229, 1993.

10. **Rivenson, A., Hoffmann, D., Prokopczyk, B., Amin, S., and Hecht, S. S.,** Induction of lung and exocrine pancreas tumors in F344 rats by tobacco-specific and Areca-derived N-nitrosamines, *Cancer Res.,* 48, 6912, 1988.

11. **Morse, M. A., Eklind, K. I., Toussaint, M., Amin, S. G., and Chung, F.-L.,** Characterization of a glucuronide metabolite of 4-(methylnitrosamino)-1-(3-pyridyl)-1-butanone (NNK) and its dose-dependent excretion in the urine of mice and rats, *Carcinogenesis,* 11, 1819, 1990.

12. **Schulze, J., Richter, E., Binder, U., and Zwickenpflug, W.,** Biliary excretion of 4-(methylnitrosamino)-1-(3-pyridyl)-1-butanone in the rat, *Carcinogenesis,* 13, 1961, 1992.

13. **Desai, D., Kagan, S. S., Amin, S., Carmella, S. G., and Hecht, S. S.,** Identification of 4-(methylnitrosamino)-1-[3-(6-hydroxypyridyl)]-1-butanone as a urinary metabolite of NNK in the rat, *Chem. Res. Toxicol.,* 6, 794, 1993.

14. **Peterson, L. A., Ng, D. K., Stearns, R. A., and Hecht, S. S.,** Formation of NADP(H) analogs of tobacco specific nitrosamines in rat liver and pancreatic microsomes, *Chem. Res. Toxicol.,* 7, 599, 1994.

15. **Murphy, S. E., Spina, D. A., Nunes, M. G., and Pullo, D. A.,** Glucuronidation of 4-(hydroxymethyl)nitrosamino-1-(3-pyridyl)-1-butanone, a metabolically activated form of 4-(methylnitrosamino)-1-(3-pyridyl)-1-butanone (NNK), by phenobarbital treated rats, *Chem. Res. Toxicol.,* 8, 772, 1995.

16. **Wiench, K., Frie, E., Schroth, P., and Wiessler, M.,** 1-C-Glucuronidation of N-nitrosodiethylamine and N-nitrosomethyl-n-pentylamine *in vivo* and in primary hepato-

cytes from rats pretreated with inducers, *Carcinogenesis,* 13, 867, 1992.

17. **Carmella, S. G., Akerkar, S., and Hecht, S. S.,** Metabolites of the tobacco-specific nitrosamine 4-(methylnitrosamino)-1-(3-pyridyl)-1-butanone in smokers' urine, *Cancer Res.,* 53, 721, 1993.

18. **Carmella, S. G., Akerkar, S., Richie, J. P., Jr., and Hecht, S. S.,** Intraindividual and interindividual differences in metabolites of the tobacco-specific lung carcinogen 4-(methylnitrosamino)-1-(3-pyridyl)-1-butanone (NNK) in smokers' urine, *Cancer Epidemiol. Biomarkers Prev.,* 4, 635, 1995.

19. **Hecht, S. S., Carmella, S. G., Murphy, S. E., Akerkar, S., Brunnemann, K. D., and Hoffmann, D.,** A tobacco-specific lung carcinogen in the urine of men exposed to cigarette smoke, *N. Engl. J. Med.,* 329, 1543, 1993.

20. **Murphy, S. E., Carmella, S. G., Idris, A. M., and Hoffmann, D.,** Uptake and metabolism of carcinogenic levels of tobacco-specific nitrosamines by Sudanese snuff dippers, *Cancer Epidemiol. Biomarkers Prev.,* 3, 423, 1994.

21. **Devereux, T. R., Anderson, M. W., and Belinsky, S. A.,** Factors regulating activation and DNA alkylation by 4-(*N*-methyl-*N*-nitrosamino)-1-(3-pyridyl)-1-butanone and nitrosodimethylamine in rat lung and isolated lung cells, and their relationship to carcinogenicity, *Cancer Res.,* 48, 4215, 1988.

22. **Smith, T. J., Guo, Z., Thomas, P. E., and Yang, C. S.,** Kinetics and enzyme involvement in the metabolism of 4-(methylnitrosamino)-1-(3-pyridyl)-1-butanone by rat lung and nasal mucosa, *Carcinogenesis,* 13, 1409, 1992.

23. **Guo, Z., Smith, T. J., Thomas, P. E., and Yang, C. S.,** Metabolism of 4-(methylnitrosamino)-1-(3-pyridyl)-1-butanone by inducible and constitutive cytochrome P450 enzymes in rats, *Arch. Biochem. Biophys.,* 298, 279, 1992.

24. **Guo, Z., Smith, T. J., Ishizaki, H., and Yang, C. S.,** Metabolism of 4-(methylnitrosamino)-1-(3-pyridyl)-1-butanone (NNK) by cytochrome P450IIB1 in a reconstituted system, *Carcinogenesis,* 12, 2277, 1991.

25. **Lacroix, D., Desrochers, M., Castonguay, A., and Anderson, A.,** Metabolism of 4-(methylnitrosamino)-1-(3-pyridyl)-1-butanone (NNK) in human kidney epithelial cells transfected with rat CYP2B1 cDNA, *Carcinogenesis,* 14, 1639, 1993.

26. **Smith, T. J., Guo, Z., Thomas, P. E., Chung, F.-L., Morse, M. A., Eklind, K., and Yang, C. S.,** Metabolism of 4-(*N*-methyl-*N*-nitrosamino)-1-(3-pyridyl)-1-butanone in mouse lung microsomes and its inhibition by isothiocyanates, *Cancer Res.,* 50, 6817, 1990.

27. **Smith, T. J., Guo, Z., Li, C., Ning, S. M., Thomas, P. E., and Yang, C. S.,** Mechanisms of inhibition of 4-(methylnitrosamino)-1-(3-pyridyl)-1-butanone bioactivation in mouse by dietary phenethyl isothiocyanate, *Cancer Res.,* 53, 3276, 1993.

28. **Hong, J.-Y., Ding, X., Smith, T. J., Coon, M. J., and Yang, C. S.,** Metabolism of 4-(methylnitrosamino)-1-(3-pyridyl)-1-butanone (NNK), a tobacco-specific carcinogen, by rabbit nasal microsomes and cytochrome P450s NMa and NMb, *Carcinogenesis,* 13, 2141, 1992.

29. **Crespi, C. L., Penman, B. W., Gelboin, H. V., and Gonzalez, F.,** A tobacco smoke-derived nitrosamine, 4-(methylnitrosamino)-1-(3-pyridyl)-1-butanone, is activated by multiple human cytochrome P450s, including the polymorphic human cytochrome P4502D6, *Carcinogenesis,* 12, 1197, 1991.

30. **Smith, T. J., Guo, Z. Y., Gonzalez, F. J., Guengerich, F. P., Stoner, G. D., and Yang, C. S.,** Metabolism of 4-(methylnitrosamino)-1-(3-pyridyl)-1-butanone in human lung and liver microsomes and cytochromes P-450 expressed in hepatoma cells, *Cancer Res.,* 52, 1757, 1992.

31. **Penman, B. W., Reece, J., Smith, T., Yang, C. S., Gelboin, H. V., Gonzalez, F. J., and Crespi, C. L.,** Characterization of a human cell line expressing high levels of cDNA-derived CYP2D6, *Pharmacogenesis,* 3, 28, 1993.

32. **Yamazaki, H., Inui, Y., Yun, C.-H., Guengerich, F. P., and Shimada, T.,** Cytochrome P450 2E1 and 2A6 enzymes as major catalysts for metabolic activation of *N*-nitrosodialkylamines and tobacco-related ni-

trosamines in human liver microsomes, *Carcinogenesis*, 13, 1789, 1992.

33. **Tiano, H. F., Hosokawa, M., Chulada, P. C., Smith, P. B., Wang, R.-L., Gonzalez, F. J., Crespi, C. L., and Langenbach, R.,** Retroviral mediated expression of human cytochrome P450 2A6 in C3H/10T1/2 cells confers transformability by 4-(methylnitrosamino)-1-(3-pyridyl)-1-butanone (NNK), *Carcinogenesis*, 14, 1421, 1993.

34. **Nesnow, S., Beck, S., Rosenblum, S., Lasley, J., Tiano, H. F., Hosokawa, M., Crespi, C. L., and Langenbach, R.,** *N*-Nitrosodiethylamine and 4-(methylnitrosamino)-1-(3-pyridyl)-1-butanone induced morphological transformation of C3H/10T1/2CL8 cells expressing human cytochrome P450 2A6, *Mutat. Res.*, 324, 93, 1994.

35. **Yang, C. S., Yoo, J. S. H., Ishizaki, H., and Hong, J.,** Cytochorome P450IIE1: roles in nitrosamine metabolism and mechanisms of regulation, *Drug Metab. Rev.*, 22, 147, 1990.

36. **Smith, T. J., Wang, L.-D., and Yang, C. S.,** Metabolism of nitrosamines in human lung and esophageal mucosa microsomes, *Proc. Am. Assoc. Cancer Res.*, 35, 136, 1994.

37. **Castonguay, A., Tharp, R., and Hecht, S. S.,** Kinetics of DNA methylation by the tobacco specific carcinogen 4-(methylnitrosamino)-1-(3-pyridyl)-1-butanone in F344 rats, in *N-Nitroso Compounds: Occurrence, Biological Effects and Relevance to Human Cancer,* O'Neill, I. K., Von Borstel, R. C., Miller, C. T., Long, J., and Bartsch, H., Eds., International Agency for Research on Cancer, Lyon, France, 1984, 805.

38. **Hecht, S. S., Trushin, N., Castonguay, A., and Rivenson, A.,** Comparative tumorigenicity and DNA methylation in F344 rats by 4-(methylnitrosamino)-1-(3-pyridyl)-1-butanone and *N*-nitrosodimethylamine, *Cancer Res.*, 46, 498, 1986.

39. **Belinsky, S. A., White, C. M., Boucheron, J. A., Richardson, F. C., Swenberg, J. A., and Anderson, M.,** Accumulation and persistence of DNA adducts in respiratory tissue of rats following multiple administrations of the tobacco specific carcinogen 4-(*N*-methyl-*N*-nitrosamino)-1-(3-pyridyl)-1-butanone, *Cancer Res.*, 46, 1280, 1986.

40. **Hecht, S. S., Spratt, T. E., and Trushin, N.,** Evidence for 4-(3-pyridyl)-4-oxobutylation of DNA in F344 rats treated with the tobacco specific nitrosamines 4-(methylnitrosamino)-1-(3-pyridyl)-1-butanone and *N'*-nitrosonornicotine, *Carcinogenesis*, 9, 161, 1988.

41. **Hecht, S. S., Peterson, L. A., and Spratt, T. E.,** Tobacco-specific nitrosamines, in *DNA Adducts: Identification and Biological Significance,* Hemminki, K., Dipple, A., Shuker, D. E. G., Kadlubar, F. F., Segerbäck, D., and Bartsch, H., Eds., International Agency for Research on Cancer, Lyon, France, 1994, 91.

42. **Peterson, L. A., Mathew, R., Murphy, S. E., Trushin, N., and Hecht, S. S.,** In vivo and in vitro persistence of pyridyloxobutyl DNA adducts from 4-(methylnitrosamino)-1-(3-pyridyl)-1-butanone, *Carcinogenesis*, 12, 2069, 1991.

43. **Murphy, S. E., Palomino, A., Hecht, S. S., and Hoffmann, D.,** Dose-response study of DNA and hemoglobin adduct formation by 4-(methylnitrosamino)-1-(3-pyridyl)-1-butanone in F344 rats, *Cancer Res.*, 50, 5446, 1990.

44. **Trushin, N., Rivenson, A., and Hecht, S. S.,** Evidence supporting the role of DNA pyridyloxobutylation in rat nasal carcinogenesis by tobacco specific nitrosamines, *Cancer Res.*, 54, 1205, 1994.

45. **Peterson, L. A. and Hecht, S. S.,** O^6-Methylguanine is a critical determinant of 4-(methylnitrosamino)-1-(3-pyridyl)-1-butanone tumorigenesis in A/J mouse lung, *Cancer Res.*, 51, 5557, 1991.

46. **Joquera, R., Castonguay, A., and Schuller, H. M.,** DNA single-strand breaks and toxicity induced by 4-(methylnitrosamino)-1-(3-pyridyl)-1-butanone or *N*-nitrosodimethylamine in hamster and rat liver, *Carcinogenesis*, 15, 389, 1994.

47. **Demkowicz-Dobrzanski, K. and Castonguay, A.,** Comparison of DNA alkali-labile sites induced by 4-(methylnitrosamino)-1-(3-pyridyl)-1-butanone and 4-oxo-4-(3-pyridyl)butanal in rat hepatocytes, *Carcinogenesis*, 12, 2135, 1991.

48. **Alaoui-Jamali, M. A., Gagnon, R., El Alami, N., and Castonguay, A.,** Cytotoxicity, sister-chromatid exchanges and DNA single-strand

breaks induced by 4-oxo-4-(3-pyridyl)butanal, a metabolite of a tobacco-specific *N*-nitrosamine, *Mutat. Res.,* 240, 25, 1990.

49. **Chung, F.-L. and Xu, Y.,** Increased 8-hydroxydeoxyguanosine levels in lung DNA of A/J mice and F344 rats treated with the tobacco-specific nitrosamine 4-(methylnitrosamino)-1-(3-pyridyl)-1-butanone, *Carcinogenesis,* 13, 1269, 1992.

50. **Carmella, S. G. and Hecht, S. S.,** Formation of hemoglobin adducts upon treatment of F344 rats with the tobacco-specific nitrosamines 4-(methylnitrosamino)-1-(3-pyridyl)-1-butanone and *N'*-nitrosonornicotine, *Cancer Res.,* 47, 2626, 1987.

51. **Peterson, L. A., Carmella, S. G., and Hecht, S. S.,** Investigations of metabolic precursors to hemoglobin and DNA adducts of 4-(methylnitrosamino)-1-(3-pyridyl)-1-butanone, *Carcinogenesis,* 11, 1329, 1990.

52. **Carmella, S. G., Kagan, S. S., and Hecht, S. S.,** Evidence that a hemoglobin adduct of 4-(methylnitrosamino)-1-(3-pyridyl)-1-butanone is a 4-(3-pyridyl)-4-oxobutyl carboxylic acid ester, *Chem. Res. Toxicol.,* 5, 76, 1992.

53. **Carmella, S. G., Kagan, S. S., Spratt, T. E., and Hecht, S. S.,** Evaluation of cysteine adduct formation in rat hemoglobin by 4-(methylnitrosamino)-1-(3-pyridyl)-1-butanone and related compounds, *Cancer Res.,* 50, 5453, 1990.

54. **Murphy, S. E. and Coletta, K. A.,** Two type of 4-(methylnitrosamino)-1-(3-pyridyl)-1-butanone hemoglobin adducts, from metabolites which migrate into or are formed in red blood cells, *Cancer Res.,* 53, 777, 1993.

55. **Mustonen, R. and Hemminki, K.,** 7-Methylguanine levels in DNA of smokers' and nonsmokers' total white blood cells, granulocytes and lymphocytes, *Carcinogenesis,* 13, 1951, 1992.

56. **Mustonen, R., Schoket, B., and Hemminki, K.,** Smoking-related DNA adducts: ^{32}P-postlabeling analysis of 7-methylguanine in human bronchial and lymphocyte DNA, *Carcinogenesis,* 14, 151, 1993.

57. **Foiles, P. G., Miglietta, L. M., Akerkar, S. A., Everson, R. B., and Hecht, S. S.,** Detection of *O*[6]-methyldeoxyguanosine in human placental DNA, *Cancer Res.,* 48, 4184, 1988.

58. **Foiles, P. G., Akerkar, S. A., Carmella, S. G., Kagan, M., Stoner, G. D., Resau, J. H., and Hecht, S. S.,** Mass spectrometric analysis of tobacco-specific nitrosamine-DNA adducts in smokers and nonsmokers, *Chem. Res. Toxicol.,* 4, 364, 1991.

59. **Carmella, S. G., Kagan, S. S., Kagan, M., Foiles, P. G., Palladino, G., Quart, A. M., Quart, E., and Hecht, S. S.,** Mass spectrometric analysis of tobacco-specific nitrosamine hemoglobin adducts in snuff dippers, smokers, and non-smokers, *Cancer Res.,* 50, 5438, 1990.

60. **Hecht, S. S., Carmella, S. G., and Murphy, S. E.,** Tobacco-specific nitrosamine hemoglobin adducts, *Methods Enzymol.,* 231, 657, 1994.

61. **Hecht, S. S., Carmella, S. G., Foiles, P. G., Murphy, S. E., and Peterson, L. A.,** Tobacco-specific nitrosamine adducts: studies in laboratory animals and humans, *Environ. Health Perspect.,* 99, 57, 1993.

62. **Falter, B., Kutzer, C., and Richter, E.,** Biomonitoring of hemoglobin adducts: aromatic amines and tobacco-specific nitrosamines, *Clin. Invest.,* 72, 364, 1994.

63. **Belinsky, S. A., Foley, J. F., White, C. M., Anderson, M. W., and Maronpot, R. R.,** Dose-response relationship between *O*[6]-methylguanine formation in Clara cells and induction of pulmonary neoplasia in the rat by 4-(methylnitrosamino)-1-(3-pyridyl)-1-butanone, *Cancer Res.,* 50, 3772, 1990.

64. **Belinsky, S. A., Dolan, M. E., White, C. M., Maronpot, R. R., Pegg, A. E., and Anderson, M. W.,** Cell specific differences in *O*[6]-methylguanine-DNA methyltransferase activity and removal of *O*[6]-methylguanine in rat pulmonary cells, *Carcinogenesis,* 9, 2053, 1988.

65. **Hecht, S. S., Lin, D., Castonguay, A., and Rivenson, A.,** Effects of α-deuterium substitution on the tumorigenicity of 4-(methylnitrosamino)-1-(3-pyridyl)-1-butanone in F344 rats, *Carcinogenesis,* 8, 291, 1987.

66. **Hecht, S. S., Lin, D., and Castonguay, A.,** Effects of α-deuterium substitution on the

mutagenicity of 4-(methylnitrosamino)-1-(3-pyridyl)-1-butanone (NNK), *Carcinogenesis,* 4, 305, 1983.

67. **Foiles, P. G., Peterson, L. A., Miglietta, L. M., and Ronai, Z.,** Analysis of mutagenic activity and ability to induce replication of polyoma DNA sequences by different model compounds of the carcinogenic tobacco-specific nitrosamine 4-(methylnitrosamino)-1-(3-pyridyl)-1-butanone, *Mutat. Res.,* 279, 91, 1992.

68. **Peterson, L. A., Liu, X.-K., and Hecht, S. S.,** Pyridyloxobutyl DNA adducts inhibit the repair of O^6-methylguanine, *Cancer Res.,* 53, 2780, 1993.

69. **Belinsky, S. A., Walker, V. E., Maronpot, R. R., Swenberg, J. A., and Anderson, M. W.,** Molecular dosimetry of DNA adduct formation and cell toxicity in rat nasal mucosa following exposure to the tobacco specific nitrosamine 4-(*N*-methyl-*N*-nitrosamino)-1-(3-pyridyl)-1-butanone and their relationship to induction of neoplasia, *Cancer Res.,* 47, 6058, 1987.

70. **Liu, L., Castonguay, A., and Gerson, S. L.,** Lack of correlation between DNA methylation and hepatocarcinogenesis in rats and hamsters treated with 4-(methylnitrosamino)-1-(3-pyridyl)-1-butanone, *Carcinogenesis,* 13, 2137, 1992.

71. **Van Benthen, J., Feron, V. J., Leeman, W. R., Wilmer, J. W. G. M., Vermeulen, E., den Engelse, L., and Scherer, E.,** Immunocytochemical identification of DNA adducts, O^6-methylguanine and 7-methylguanine, in respiratory and other tissues of rat, mouse and Syrian hamster exposed to 4-(methylnitrosamino)-1-(3-pyridyl)-1-butanone, *Carcinogenesis,* 15, 2023, 1994.

72. **Hecht, S. S., Jordan, K. G., Choi, C.-I., and Trushin, N.,** Effects of deuterium substitution on the tumorigenicity of 4-(methylnitrosamino)-1-(3-pyridyl)-1-butanone and 4-(methyl-nitrosamino)-1-(3-pyridyl)-1-butanol in A/J mice, *Carcinogenesis,* 11, 1017, 1990.

73. **Belinsky, S. A., Devereux, T. R., Foley, J. F., Maronpot, R. R., and Anderson, M. W.,** Role of the alveolar type II cell in the devel-opment and progression of pulmonary tumors induced by 4-(methylnitrosamino)-1-(3-pyridyl)-1-butanone in the A/J mouse, *Cancer Res.,* 52, 3164, 1992.

74. **Devereux, T. R., Anderson, M. W., and Belinsky, S. A.,** Role of *ras* protooncogene activation in the formation of spontaneous and nitrosamine-induced lung tumors in the resistant C3H mouse, *Carcinogenesis,* 12, 299, 1991.

75. **Devereux, T. R., Belinsky, S. A., Maronpot, R. R., White, C. M., Hegi, M. E., Patel, A. C., Foley, J. F., Greenwell, A., and Anderson, M. W.,** Comparison of pulmonary O^6-methylguanine DNA adduct levels and Ki-*ras* activation in lung tumors from resistant and susceptible mouse strains, *Mol. Carcinogen.,* 8, 177, 1993.

76. **Belinsky, S. A., Devereux, T. R., Maronpot, R. R., Stoner, G. D., and Anderson, M. W.,** The relationship between the formation of promutagenic adducts and the activation of the K-ras proto-oncogene in lung tumors from A/J mice treated with nitrosamines, *Cancer Res.,* 49, 5305, 1989.

77. **Ronai, Z., Gradia, S., Peterson, L. A., and Hecht, S. S.,** G to A transitions and G to T transversions in codon 12 of the Ki-*ras* oncogene isolated from mouse lung tumors induced by 4-(methylnitrosamino)-1-(3-pyridyl)-1-butanone (NNK) and related DNA methylating and pyridyloxobutylating agents, *Carcinogenesis,* 14, 2419, 1993.

78. **Matzinger, S. A., Gunning, W. T., You, M., and Castonguay, A.,** Ki-*ras* mutations in 4-(methylnitrosamino)-1-(3-pyridyl)-1-butanone-initiated and butylated hydroxytoluene-promoted lung tumors in A/J mice, *Mol. Carcinogen.,* 11, 42, 1994.

79. **Chen, B., Liu, L., Castonguay, A., Maronpot, R. R., Anderson, M. W., and You, M.,** Dose-dependent *ras* mutation spectra in *N*-nitrosodiethylamine induced mouse liver tumors and 4-(methylnitrosamino)-1-(3-pyridyl)-1-butanone induced mouse lung tumors, *Carcinogenesis,* 14, 1603, 1993.

80. **Oreffo, V. I. C., Lin, H.-W., Padmanabhan, R., and Witschi, H.,** K-*ras* and *p53* point

mutations in 4-(methylnitrosamino)-1-(3-pyridyl)-1-butanone-induced hamster lung tumors, *Carcinogenesis,* 14, 451, 1993.

81. **Belinsky, S. A., Devereux, T. R., White, C. M., Foley, J. F., Maronpot, R. R., and Anderson, M. W.,** Role of Clara cells and type II cells in the development of pulmonary tumors in rats and mice following exposure to a tobacco-specific nitrosamine, *Exp. Lung Res.,* 17, 263, 1991.

82. **Rodenhuis, S. and Slebos, R. J. C.,** Clinical significance of ras oncogene activation in human lung cancer, *Cancer Res. [Suppl.],* 52, 2665s, 1992.

83. **Hecht, S. S., Chen, C. B., Ohmori, T., and Hoffmann, D.,** Comparative carcinogenicity in F344 rats of the tobacco specific nitrosamines, *N'*-nitrosonornicotine and 4-(*N*-methyl-*N*-nitrosamino)-1-(3-pyridyl)-1-butanone, *Cancer Res.,* 40, 298, 1980.

EPIDEMIOLOGY OF CANCER BY TOBACCO PRODUCTS AND THE SIGNIFICANCE OF TSNA

THE BIOLOGICAL SIGNIFICANCE OF TOBACCO-SPECIFIC *N*-NITROSAMINES: SMOKING AND ADENOCARCINOMA OF THE LUNG

Critical Reviews in Toxicology, 26(2):183–198 (1996)

Epidemiology of Cancer by Tobacco Products and the Significance of TSNA

Prakash C. Gupta, P. R. Murti, and R. B. Bhonsle

International Agency for Research on Cancer, Lyon and Basic Dental Research Unit, and WHO Collaborating Centre for Oral Cancer Prevention, Tata Institute of Fundamental Research, Bombay, India

ABSTRACT: Globally, oral cancer is one of the ten common cancers. In some parts of the world, including the Indian subcontinent, oral cancer is a major cancer problem. Tobacco use is the most important risk factor for oral cancer. The most common form of tobacco use, cigarette smoking, demonstrates a very high relative risk — in a recent cohort study (CPS II), even higher than lung cancer. In areas where tobacco is used in a smokeless form, oral cancer incidence is generally high. In the West, especially in the U.S. and Scandinavia, smokeless tobacco use consists of oral use of snuff. In Central, South, and Southeast Asia smokeless tobacco use encompasses *nass, naswar, khaini, mawa, mishri, gudakhu,* and betel quid. In India tobacco is smoked in many ways; the most common is *bidi,* others being *chutta,* including reverse smoking, *hooka,* and clay pipe. A voluminous body of research data implicating most of these forms of tobacco use emanates from the Indian subcontinent. These studies encompass case and case-series reports, and case-control, cohort, and intervention studies. Collectively, the evidence fulfills the epidemiological criteria of causality: strength, consistency, temporality, and coherence. The biological plausibility is provided by the identification of several carcinogens in tobacco, the most abundant and strongest being tobacco-specific *N*-nitrosamines such as *N*-nitrosonornicotine (NNN) and 4-(methylnitrosamino)-1-(3-pyridyl)-1-butanone (NNK). These are formed by *N*-nitrosation of nicotine, the major alkaloid responsible for addiction to tobacco. The etiological relationship between tobacco use and oral cancer has provided us with a comprehensive model for understanding carcinogenesis.

KEY WORDS: cancer, oral, etiology, smoking, tobacco, smokeless.

I. INTRODUCTION

An estimate for the year 1980 showed that there were 6.35 million incident cases of the most frequent cancers globally.[1] Of these, 49% occurred in the developed countries and 51% in the developing world, whereas the population ratio is 1:3. There are marked geographic variations in the incidence of different types of cancer all over the world, almost all of them due to differences in the extent of exposure and the type of etiological/risk factors in the respective regions. Overall, 1 to 1.5 million cancers (16 to 24%) are tobacco related, a vast majority occurring in the oral cavity, esophagus, larynx, and lung, and a fraction in such distant organs as the pancreas, cervix, bladder, and kidney.

A classic example of tobacco-related cancer in the developed world is lung cancer. It is the most common cause of cancer death in the U.S.; about 90% of deaths among men and 79% among women can be directly attributed to cigarette smoking.[2] Oral cancer, with an attributable risk of 91% for tobacco use,[3] is the most important tobacco-related cancer in some parts of the developing world, especially Southeast Asia.

Oral cancer is the sixth most common cancer in the world,[4] with over 50% of the estimated 412,000 incident cases occurring in the developing world. There is an increasing trend in its incidence and mortality in Western populations;[5–7] about 262,000 deaths are estimated to occur due to this disease.[7] Compared with Western countries, the problem of oral cancer is more serious in India, where 10% of the estimated 644,600 new cancers that develop annually are oral cancers.[8] Extensive epidemiological data implicating tobacco as an etiological factor for oral cancer are available from Southeast Asia as well as the rest of the world. The epidemiological data are well supported by laboratory findings about the chemical carcinogens in tobacco and the mechanism of carcinogenesis. In this article we appraise the etiological role of tobacco in cancer using oral cancer as a model for evaluating a variety of data.

A major advantage in using oral cancer as a model is that whereas the only data available for the relationship between other cancers and tobacco use is for cigarette smoking, for oral cancer, in addition to cigarette smoking, a considerable amount of data are available about other forms of tobacco use as well.

II. TOBACCO USE AND CARCINOGENIC CONSTITUENTS

Since the introduction of tobacco to the Old World in 1492, its use spread with remarkable rapidity to all sections of the society and geographic locations. No country today is tobacco free. Currently, the oral use of tobacco is practiced in diverse smoked and smokeless forms.[9–12] In the U.S., some 4.9 million adult males use smokeless tobacco[13] and in 1985, 56 million people in the age range of 15 to 84 years smoke cigarettes.[2] According to one estimate, of the 400 million adults aged 15 years and over in India, 189 million (47%) use tobacco in one form or another.[14] According to a WHO estimate,[15] 65% of men use tobacco (43% smoke and 30% chew) compared with 33% of women (4% smoke and 30% chew tobacco).

The pattern of tobacco use varies a great deal between Southeast Asia and other countries. The most common, in fact, often the only form of tobacco use in most parts of the world, is cigarette smoking. Although cigarettes are becoming increasingly more popular in Southeast Asia, several indigenous preparations are used for smoking: viz. *bidi*, *chutta*, *dhumti*, clay pipe, *hookah*, *keeyos*, and *kreteks*. Smokeless tobacco use is even more diverse. It is used for chewing (in betel quid, *mawa*, *ghutka*, *pan masala*, *shamma*, etc.), keeping in the mouth for sucking (*khaini*, *zarda*, *nass* and *naswar*), and for application over teeth and gums (*mishri*, *gudhaku*, *bajjar*, dry snuff, and creamy snuff).

Most products used for smoking are prepared from *Nicotiana tabacum*, and for smokeless tobacco use, from *N. rustica*. Of the several thousand chemical constituents recognized in both forms of tobacco, a number of them have been identified as toxic, tumorigenic, and carcinogenic.[16–20] In addition to PAH (polynuclear aromatic hydrocarbons), the most important and abundant carcinogenic agents in tobacco are the tobacco-specific *N*-nitrosamines (TSNA), namely, NNN (nitrosonornicotine) and NNK (4-(methylnitrosamino)-1-(3-pyridyl)-1-butanone). These are the likely causative agents for oral cancer among smokers as well as smokeless tobacco users[21] (Table 1). Their levels in various tobacco products, however, exhibit wide variations[19,22] (Tables 2 to 4).

TABLE 1
Probable Causative Agents in Tobacco Carcinogenesis

Cancer site	TSNA	Other tumor initiators and carcinogens	Tumor-enhancing factors
Oral cavity, snuff dippers	NNN, NNK	^{210}Po (?), Aldehydes	HSV-1 and HSV-2, nutrition, physical irritation
Smokers	NNN, NNK	^{210}Po (?)	HSV-1 and HSV-2, nutrition, alcohol
Lungs, smokers	NNK, NNAL	PAH, ^{210}Po, (minor) volatile aldehydes, 1,3-butadiene (?), Cr, Cd, Ni (?)	Tumor promoters and cocarcinogens, aldehydes
Esophagus, smokers	NNK, NNB	Volatile *N*-nitrosamines (?)	Catechols, alcohol
Pancreas, smokers	NNK, NNAL		Nutrition
Bladder, smokers		4-Amino-biphenyl, 2-naphthylamine, 2-toluidine, other aromatic amines (?)	Infectious agents (?)

From Hoffmann, D., Rivenson, A., Fung-Lung, C., and Hecht, H. H., *CRC Crit. Rev. Toxicol.*, 21, 305, 1991.

III. TOBACCO USE AND ORAL CANCER

A link between the use of smokeless tobacco and cancer was suspected as early as 1761 in the U.S.,[23] and a case report implicating snuff dipping with oral cancer appeared in 1915.[24] From India, descriptions of the relationship between tobacco use, mainly betel quid chewing, and oral cancer abound since the turn of this century,[25–27] with the first case-control study in 1933.[28] Since then, a variety of information has become available from case reports, case series, and descriptive, case-control, cross-sectional, pro-spective, and interventional studies. For a long time there was confusion about the etiological role of so-called "betel nut" and tobacco in oral cancer. A review of the literature in 1982 established that it was tobacco, rather than areca nut in the betel quid, that was responsible for most oral cancers in the region.[29] Later reviews confirmed these findings and further pinpointed the importance of tobacco in oral cancer.[2,9,10,30–32]

A. Smoking and Oral Cancer

As mentioned earlier, tobacco is smoked in many forms, and among them habits of

TABLE 2
TSNA in Smokeless Tobacco, 1981 to 1989

Country and Tobacco Type	Samples (n)	NNM[a] (μg/g)	NAT[a] (μg/g)	NAB[a] (μg/g)	NNK[a] (μg/g)
U.S.					
Moist snuff	16	0.83–64.00	0.24–215.00	0.01–6.70	0.08–8.30
Chewing tobacco	2	0.67–1.50	0.7–2.4[b]	0.11–0.38	
Dry snuff	6	9.4–55.0	11–40	0.5–1.2	0.88–14.00
Sweden					
Moist snuff	8	2.0–6.1	0.9–2.4	0.04–0.14	0.61–1.70
Canada					
Moist snuff	2	50–79	152–170	4.0–4.8	3.2–5.8
Plug	1	2.1	1.7[b]		0.24
Germany					
Plug	2	1.4–2.1	0.36–0.55		0.03–0.04
Nasal snuff	7	2.8–19	1.0–5.8		0.58–6.40
India					
Chewing tobacco	4	0.47–0.85	0.40–0.50[b]		0.13–0.23
Zarda	11	0.40–79.00	0.78–99[b]		0.22–24.00
U.S.S.R.					
Nass	4	0.12–0.52	0.04–0.33		0.02–0.11
U.K.					
Moist snuff	7	1.1–52.0	2.0–65.0[b]		0.4–13.0
Nasal snuff	5	3.0–16.0	1.8–2.5[b]		0.97–4.30

[a] NNN, *N*′-nitrosonornicotine; NAT, *N*′-nitrosoanatabine; NAB, *N*′-nitrosoanabasine; NNK, 4-(methylnitrosamino)-1-(3-pyridyl)-1-butanone.
[b] Contains NAB.

From Brunnemann, K. D. and Hoffmann, D., in Smokeless Tobacco or Health, an International Perspective, NIH Publ. No. 92-3461, U.S. Department of Health and Human Services, Public Health Service, National Institutes of Health, 1992, 96.

TABLE 3
TSNA in Tobacco and Betel Quid with Tobacco

Tobacco species	Betel quid	TSNA (μg/g dry wt)		
		NNN	NNK	NAT + NAB
N. Tabacum	–	1.50	0.52	1.30
N. Rustica	–	14.96	25.77	78.17
N. Rustica	+	26.80	4.90	ND

[a] ND, not done.

From Bhide, S. V., Kulkami, J. R., Padma, P. R., Amonkar, A. J., Maru, G. B., Nair, U. J., and Nair, J., Studies on tobacco specific nitrosamines and other carcinogenic agents in smokeless tobacco products, in *Tobacco and Health, The Indian Scene,* Sanghvi, L. D. and Notani, P. N., Eds., Tata Memorial Centre, Bombay, 1989, 121.

TABLE 4
TSNA in Indian Tobacco Used in Cigarettes, *Bidi*, and *Chutta*

Type	Sample	TSNA (µg/g)		
		NNN	NAT	NNK
Cigarette	1	58.0	15.1	4.8
	2	1.3	8.8	0.4
Bidi	1	6.2	9.0	0.4
	2	12.0	12.5	1.4
Chutta	1	295.8	686.7	210.3

From Bhide, S. V., Kulkami, J. R., Padma, P. R., Amonkar, A. J., Maru, G. B., Nair, U. J., and Nair, J., Studies on tobacco specific nitrosamines and other carcinogenic agents in smokeless tobacco products, in *Tobacco and Health, The Indian Scene,* Sanghvi, L. D. and Notani, P. N., Eds., Tata Memorial Centre, Bombay, 1989, 121.

cigarette, *bidi*, reverse *chutta*, cigar, and pipe smoking have been studied for their relationship with oral cancer. Smoking is the strongest risk factor for pharyngeal cancers as well, and in some publications the combined data for two types of cancers are available.

1. Cigarette Smoking

Cigarette smoking is an important etiologic factor for oral cancer, reported since the earliest studies, and detailed reviews are available on this topic.[10,30] Risk estimates seem to have increased over time. For example, in Cancer Prevention Study I (CPS I) (25 states, 1959–1965) in the U.S., the relative risk estimates for current cigarette smokers for oral/pharyngeal cancer for men and women were 6.33 and 1.96, respectively, while the corresponding risks in CPS II (50 states, 1982 to 1986) were 27.48 and 5.59.[2] While in CPS I the risk for oral/pharyngeal cancers ranked third among men, next only to lung (11.35) and larynx (10.00), in CPS II it ranked first, followed by lung (22.36) and larynx (10.48). From CPS I data, 74% of deaths from oral/pharyngeal cancers for men and 27% for women could be attributed to cigarette smoking, whereas in CPS II they increased to 92 and 61%, respectively.

The relative risk (RR) for oral cancer due to smoking seems to be high in Brazil, where the incidence also is reported as high.[33,34] In a case-control study of 232 oral cancers (ICD = 141+143 to 145) and 464 controls, the effect of tobacco, alcohol, diet, oral hygiene, and other factors was studied using a multivariate analysis.[34] The RR for cigarette smoking (adjusted for alcohol consumption) was 6.3, and that for hand-rolled cigarettes (black tobacco) was 7.0. Compared with a baseline of 1.0 for a life-time consumption of <1 pack per year, the RR for >100 packs per year was 14.8. Habit cessation decreased the RR from 9.3 in current smokers, to 2.9 in ex-smokers following 1 to 10 years of cessation and became insignificant after 10 years of discontinuation. The risks in those who smoked hand-rolled cigarettes also declined from 14.4 in current smokers to 2.3 in those who quit smoking for >10 years.

In a study of 57 cases of tongue cancer and 353 controls from Uruguay,[35] the RR for current cigarette smokers was 29.4 and that for ex-smokers was 11.8. Compared with those who started smoking after 20 years of age, the RR was 2.0 for those who started smoking before 14 years of age. A strong dose-response relationship was also observed, compared with those smoking <10 cigarettes per day, the RR was 5.2 for those smoking 31+ cigarettes a day. Likewise, compared with those who had smoked for <29 years, the RR was 3.6 for those who smoked for over 50 years. Conversely, compared with current smokers, cessation of the habit resulted in a risk reduction to 0.2 in those who quit smoking for more than 10 years. Considering smoking of blond tobacco as a baseline, the RR was 4.0 for smoking black tobacco and 1.8 for mixed tobaccos. Black tobacco smoke was shown to contain a higher concentration of *N*-nitroso compounds and aromatic amines with a high alkalinity, perhaps accounting for a higher risk.

In a study of 122 oropharyngeal cancers and 606 controls from Italy, a four- to six-fold increase in risk with medium to high tobacco consumption was observed.[36] The risks increased with duration and were higher when the onset of smoking began early; conversely, they decreased with the cessation of smoking. The population attributable risks in this study were 72% among men and 54% among women. In another study of 439 oropharyngeal cancers and 2106 controls from Italy, smoking accounted for 81 to 87% of oral cancer in males and 42 to 47% in females using different modeling procedures.[37]

2. Bidi *Smoking*

Bidi is a 4 to 7.5-cm-long cheap smoking stick made by rolling a dried, rectangular piece of *temburni* leaf (*Diospyros melanoxylon*) with 0.15 to 0.25 g of sun-dried, flaked tobacco into a conical shape and securing the roll with a thread. An estimated 136 million of the 400 million adults in India smoke this product.[14] It is also popular in Pakistan, Sri Lanka, Bangladesh, and several other countries in Southeast Asia.

The relationship between *bidi* smoking and oral cancer can be ascertained from a variety of epidemiological data. In a cross-sectional survey in India, the prevalence of oral cancer was 0.57 per 1000 in bidi smokers compared with 0.18 in nonusers of tobacco and 1.56 in those who smoked and drank alcohol.[38] A case-control study of 725 cases and 440 controls from India and Sri Lanka demonstrated relative risks for smokers to be significant (2.1 for men and 11.5 for women).[39] In a study of 411 cases and controls from Bombay, the relative risk for *bidi* smoking was 2.8.[40] A case-control study from Pakistan showed the RR for *bidi* smoking to be 36.[41] A recent case-control study of

228 tongue and floor of the mouth cancers and 453 controls from India showed that *bidi* smoking alone was an independent risk factor and that there was a strong dose-response relationship;[42] the highest risk, however, was observed in those who smoked both *bidis* and cigarettes. In contrast, another study of 348 oral cancer cases and an equal number of controls in India showed a lower but significant risk (1.4) for *bidi* smoking.[43] A cohort study in India reported the incidence of oral cancer to be 39 per 100,000 among smokers (predominantly *bidi*) compared with zero among nonusers of tobacco.[44] The target sites for *bidi* smoking were reported to be the posterior locations of the mouth such as the oropharynx and posterior aspect of the tongue.[39,40,45]

Experimental studies showed that *bidi* smoke contains several toxic and mutagenic substances and TSNA that are demonstrated as carcinogenic. *Bidi* contains a smaller amount of tobacco (0.15 to 0.25 g) than a cigarette (1 g) [12] and produces a smaller volume of smoke;[46,47] yet, it delivers 45 to 50 mg of tar[16] compared with 18 to 28 mg in an Indian cigarette.[48] Compared with U.S. cigarettes, the mainstream smoke of *bidi* contains much higher concentrations of several toxic agents such as hydrogen cyanide (903 vs. 445 µg), carbon monoxide (7.7 vs. 3.5 vol%), ammonia (284 vs 180 µg), other volatile phenols (264 vs. 174 µg), and carcinogenic hydrocarbons such as benz[*a*] anthracene (117 vs. 81 ng) and benz[*o*]pyrene (78 vs. 47 ng).[16] *Bidis* also deliver more nicotine (1.74 to 2.05 mg) than Indian cigarettes (1.55 to 1.92 mg).[48] The NNN and NNK levels of *bidi* tobacco ranged from 6.2 to 12 µg/g compared with 1.3 to 58.0 µg/g in cigarette tobacco.[19] *Bidi* smoke condensate was shown to induce carcinomas in experimental animals.[49]

3. *Reverse* Chutta *Smoking*

Chutta is a coarsely prepared cheroot made by rolling tobacco leaf into a cylindrical shape, one end of which is tied with a thread.[12] In some districts in the states of Andhra Pradesh and Orissa along the east coast of India, it is often smoked in reverse, that is, with the lighted end inside the mouth, mostly by women.

Reverse *chutta* smoking causes squamous cell carcinoma of the palate, which otherwise is a rare location for cancer. In the Visakhapatnam district where this habit is widely prevalent, the frequency of palatal cancer in a hospital was 38 to 48%,[50,51] while in other areas in India it was 3 to 12%.[52–55] In a 10-year cohort study in the neighboring Srikakulam district where reverse smoking is equally widespread, the annual age-adjusted incidence rate of palatal cancer was 21 per 100,000, and it was exclusively seen in reverse smokers (37 per 100,000).[56]

Chutta tobacco contains very high levels of TSNA–NNN (295.8 μ/g), NNK (210.3 μ/g), and NAT (686.7 μ/g) (Table 4). During reverse smoking, the palatal mucosa is exposed to the pyrolyzed products of tobacco, and the intense heat increases its temperature to 58°C. Application of *chutta* smoke condensate in acetone to the skin of Swiss mice and albino rats followed by exposure to heat resulted in skin cancers in 79% of the 14 animals. In contrast, no cancer developed in an untreated group, a group treated with tobacco tar alone, or a group given heat alone.[57] The investigators opined that heat functioned as a cocarcinogen and accelerated neoplastic change.

4. Miscellaneous Smoking Habits

In the U.S., pipe and cigar smoking is indicated as a causal factor for oral cancer.[30] The mortality ratios for cancers of the larynx, oral cavity, and esophagus are similar for smokers whether they smoke cigars, pipes, or cigarettes.[2]

Considering nonsmokers as a reference category, the Brazilian study[34] showed a slightly higher relative risk of 19.4 in "ever"

cigar smokers compared with 16.4 in "never" cigar smokers for tongue cancer. Overall, pipe smoking showed a much higher risk (13.9 for "ever" smokers) compared with individuals who never smoked pipes (6.4).

B. Smokeless Tobacco Use and Oral Cancer

1. Western Forms

In Western countries, smokeless tobacco is used in the form of chewing tobacco (in the U.S., plug, roll, or twist), snuff dipping (moist or dry), and recently as portion-packed in teabags such as sachets containing moist snuff. Several case-control studies demonstrated high relative risk estimates,[58–60] and a strong dose-response relationship[61] between smokeless tobacco use and oral/pharyngeal cancer. In a review, it was concluded that there was "sufficient" evidence that smokeless tobacco use is carcinogenic to humans.[9] Additional information from three recent studies shows that oral cancer risks were elevated among users of smokeless tobacco with relative risks ranging from 2.3 to 11.2, confirming earlier evaluations.[62]

2. Betel Quid with Tobacco

In many countries in Southeast Asia and in emigrant populations from this area, the habit of chewing betel quid is widespread. An estimated 200 million people chew betel quid all over the world.[9] Betel quid contains four main ingredients: betel leaf (*Piper betle*), areca nut (*Areca catechu*), slaked lime (Ca(OH)$_2$), and, most often, tobacco. There are, nevertheless, wide regional variations in the ingredients used and the mechanics of chewing.[11,12] Several varieties of tobacco that contain high levels of TSNA (Tables 2 and 3) are used in betel quid, thereby exposing the oral mucosa of a chewer to these carcinogenic agents. In addition to TSNA, due to the inclusion of areca nut, a betel quid chewer is exposed to arecoline-derived nitrosamines, the most powerful of which are 3-(methylnitrosamino) propionitrile (MNPN) and 3-(methylnitrosamino) propionaldehyde (MNPA).[63] The evidence linking betel quid chewing and oral cancer is extensive, and it confirms the epidemiological concept of the causality of association. Therefore, for this habit, the data are reviewed in an approximate hierarchy of strength of epidemiologic evidence.

a. Ecological Observations

This is the earliest form of observation linking betel quid chewing with oral cancer. It refers to the observation of a high frequency of oral cancer in areas where betel quid chewing is widespread.[26,27] The differences in the incidence of oral cancer and tobacco usage in different ethnic groups also constitute ecological evidence. For example, the incidence of oral cancer among Parsees, a community that does not generally indulge in smoking or chewing tobacco, was estimated to be about one fifth of the incidence in the general population.[64] A similar example is that in Malaysia, oral cancer was more common in the Indian community (relative frequency of 33.6%) than in the Malays (relative frequency of 9.5%), and Indians usually chewed betel quid with tobacco, whereas Malays did not include tobacco in the quid.[65] The ecological observations constitute rather weak evidence for inferring a causal association.

b. Frequency of Chewing Habits Among Oral Cancer Patients

The high frequency of betel quid chewing among oral cancer patients observed in several descriptive studies indicates that despite the absence of controls, tobacco usage could be incriminated. Paymaster (1962) reported that 81% of 4212 oral cancer patients used tobacco, and of these 36% were chewers, 23% smokers, and 22% practiced both chewing and smoking.[66] Similar observations have been made by several investigators in other areas in India and outside. The observation that the site of origin of oral cancer corresponds to the area of placement of tobacco quid[39] is also strong evidence in favor of the role of betel quid chewing in oral cancer. Such evidence is supportive, but may not be sufficient for inferring a causal association.

c. Evidence from Case-Control Studies

Case-control studies provide the RR estimates. In Thailand, the RR estimate for betel quid chewing was significant for both men (2.3) and women (3.2) using multivariate regression analysis to adjust for confounding variables.[67] In Pakistan, the RR for betel quid chewing among men and women was 8.1 and 14.1, respectively.[41] In India, the crude RR for betel quid chewing habits in several studies[9] ranged from 7.6 to 27.0, and all of these were highly significant. In a more recent study of 348 oral cancer cases and an equal number of controls, the RR for chewing betel quid with tobacco was 14.6.[43] In a series of studies from Trivandrum, India, risk factors for cancers of the various parts of the oral cavity were evaluated with 228 cases of cancer of the tongue and the floor of the mouth, 414 cases of cancers of the buccal and labial mucosae, 187 cases of gingival cancers, and a large number of controls.[42,68,69] In each study, chewing of betel quid with tobacco emerged as the strongest risk factor.

d. Evidence from Cross-Sectional Studies

Cross-sectional, population-based studies[70,71] provide the data for the prevalence of oral cancer among people with and without tobacco habits. In these studies from India, among over 150,000 individuals, although there was a substantial number of non-habitues, 14 of the 38 oral cancers occurred in people who were solely betel quid chewers, 24 among other tobacco users, and none among nonusers of tobacco.

e. Evidence from Prospective Studies

Prospective studies provide the incidence rates of oral cancer among people with and without tobacco habits on the basis of the follow-up of cohorts. In the most extensive study of its kind in India, 30,000 individuals were followed-up over a 10-year period in three areas.[56] The betel-quid chewing habit was common in Ernakulam, and the annual age-adjusted incidence of oral cancer was 23 per 100,000 among betel quid chewers vs. zero among nonhabitues. In another study from Ahmedabad, in a 2-year follow-up period, the annual age-adjusted incidence of oral cancer among chewers was 31 per 100,000 vs. zero among nonusers.[44]

f. Dose-Response Relationship

The dose-response relationship provides evidence of the trend of the association between the extent of exposure to the etiological agent (the dose) and the risk of oral cancer. This was first demonstrated for betel quid chewing by Orr[28] in 1933. In 1966, Hirayama[39] reported a RR of 8.4 when the frequency of chewing per day, was less than two, 17.6 when the frequency rose to six or more, and 63 when the quid was retained in the mouth while asleep. In a recent study,[43] the dose-response relationship of duration, frequency, and retaining the quid in the mouth while sleeping showed an increase in RR with an increase in each parameter. In the series of studies from Trivandrum, the dose-response relationship was significant using frequency per day, duration in years, and chewing years (product of frequency and duration) as markers of dose.[42,68,69] The dose-response relationship remained significant after including other possible risk factors (smoking, alcohol, and snuff inhalation) in stepwise regression analyses.

g. Evidence from Intervention Studies

A prospective intervention study demonstrated a decrease in the risk of oral cancer following a reduction in tobacco usage. In this study of 36,000 tobacco users, including a large proportion of betel quid chewers, intensive health education regarding the oral health effects of tobacco use was given to all individuals. After 1 year, this resulted in some individuals stopping and a considerable number reducing their tobacco use, leading to a significantly higher regression rate of leukoplakia among these individuals compared with those who did not stop or reduce their habits.[72] At the end of 10 years of intervention, about 15% of men and 18% of women in the intervention cohort quit betel quid chewing compared with 2 and 8%, respectively, in the control cohort. This resulted in a drop in the annual incidence of leukoplakia among chewers to 327 per 100,000 in men and 204 per 100,000 among women in the intervention cohort from 521 and 456, respectively, in the control cohort (risk ratios of 0.63 and 0.45, respectively).[73,74] Because most oral cancers in this population developed from leukoplakia,[56] and leukoplakia was shown to be a precancerous lesion with a high RR for malignant transformation (ranging from 25.6 in homogeneous leukoplakia to 3243.2 in nodular leukoplakia),[75] these findings implied a reduction in the risk of oral cancer. Epidemiologically, this is the strongest kind of evidence possible, except, of course, for the shortcomings caused by the design limitations of the study. The shortcomings were a lack of randomization, nonconcurrence of the intervention and control cohorts, and substitution of leukoplakia as the end point in place of oral cancer.

3. Chewing Areca Nut Without Tobacco

As stated earlier, there was considerable confusion in the literature, with often quoted statements such as "the high incidence of oral cancer in India is due to betel nut chewing." The question of carcinogenecity of chewing areca nut without tobacco was addressed in an epidemiological review,[29] and it was shown that chewing betel quid without tobacco carried either an "insignificant" or a "significantly lower risk" for oral cancer compared with chewing tobacco containing quids. A dissenting note has come from South Africa, where women of Indian origin chew areca nut without tobacco and are not exposed to other risk factors such as smoking or alcohol, but show a high risk for oral cancer (RR of 43.9).[76]

A recent study of 348 oral cancer cases and an equal number of controls from India reported an RR for chewing betel quid with tobacco to be 14.6 compared with 1.7 for chewing without tobacco.[43]

4. Miscellaneous Habits

In this section we describe briefly the probable role of several other types of tobacco use, viz., tobacco-lime use (*khaini*), *nass*, *naswar*, *alshamma*, and *alqat*.

a. Tobacco-Lime Use

Placement of a mixture of tobacco and lime (known as *khaini* in North India) is widely prevalent in certain regions in India and Pakistan. Studies in India and Pakistan showed very high RRs (up to 41.2).[41,77]

b. Nass *and* Naswar *Use*

Nass is a mixture of tobacco, ash, and cotton or sesame oil, and *naswar* consists of powdered tobacco, slaked lime, indigo, cardamom oil, menthol, etc. They are used in Soviet Central Asia, Afghanistan, Iran, and Pakistan. *Nass* and *naswar* use showed high RRs (20.4 and 14.2, respectively) for oral cancer in Pakistan.[41] There is some evidence that *nass* is involved in the pathogenesis of oral cancer in Soviet Central Asia.[78]

c. Alshamma *and* Alqat *Use*

These are the traditional forms of chewable tobacco, also known as Yemeni snuff, and are popular in Yemen and in some parts of Saudi Arabia. In a case series, all 38 oral cancer patients reported using these products;[79] 42% used *shamma* alone, and 58% used both. The median duration of use of these products was 15 and 12 years, respectively. Only a few cases smoked cigarettes. In another study, all eight oral cancer patients seen over a 2-year period in the Asir region of Saudi Arabia used *shamma* for 25 years or longer.[80] *In vitro* bioassays showed *shamma* to be mutagenic.[81]

V. TSNA CARCINOGENESIS

While epidemiological data identify tobacco as the most important etiological factor for oral cancer, several experimental approaches identify TSNA as the main cancer-causing constituents in tobacco (Table 1). Studies using a variety of experimental approaches convincingly explained the mechanism of carcinogenesis of TSNA. TSNA are procarcinogens, which are metabolically activated by α-hydroxylation to form unstable α-hydroxynitrosamines. These decompose to diazohydroxides which react with cellular components, including nucleophilic centers of DNA.[20] *In vitro* assays with explants of human buccal mucosa, esophagi, bronchi, and peripheral lung have revealed that these tissues have the capability to metabolize NNK and NNN to alkyldiazohydroxides that can react with DNA.[18]

Evidence indicates[63] that arecoline, which is a major alkaloid in areca nut, also yields nitrosamines such as MNPN, MNPA, *N*-nitrosoguvacoline (NG), and *N*-nitrosoguvacine (NGC). MNPN induces benign and malignant tumors of the esophagus, tongue, nasal cavity, and liver of rats. It alkylates DNA *in vitro* and *in vivo* to 7-methulguanine, O^6-methylguanine, 7-(2-cyanoethyl) guanine, and O^6-(2-cyanoethyl)guanine. Thus, while the experimental evidence for carcinogenecity of tobacco is very strong, for the areca nut it is indicative but perhaps not yet confirmatory.

VI. SUMMARY

Carcinogenesis is a complex process that involves a causative agent and host susceptibility. This is, of course, a simplistic statement, as we know that the contribution of each of these in turn is governed by innumerable factors, known and unknown. It is estimated that, globally, tobacco is responsible for 16 to 24% of all cancers; experimental approaches have substantiated the fact that tobacco does play a vital role in carcinogenesis. Specifically, TSNA have been recognized as probable agents in tobacco for cancers in various sites in addition to other initiators, carcinogens, and enhancing factors (Table 1). It is worthwhile examining the epidemiologic evidence demonstrating the etiological role of tobacco utilizing oral cancer as a model.

In the epidemiological sense, a causal relationship between an agent and the effect can be inferred when the association shows properties of consistency, strength, temporal relationship, specificity, and coherence. A causal association can only be deduced when all the epidemiological criteria are satisfied and pathological and experimental data are supportive. The fulfillment of these parameters seems complete for oral cancer and tobacco use. The consistency of the association is clearly demonstrated, as the observations come from several investigators, diverse population groups, across different regions of the world, and over a long time span. This association is shown to be very strong as revealed by the magnitude of the RRs for a variety of tobacco uses that were all very high. An important criterion of strength is the dose-response relationship, and this was shown to be significant using the frequency of everyday use and the duration of use as markers. Another criterion of strength well demonstrated was the decrease in risk among ex-smokers and the effect of the cessation of tobacco use. The temporal nature of the association was demonstrated by the fact that the cause (i.e., tobacco use) preceded the effect (oral cancer) by many years. This was especially clear from population based studies of large cohorts with and without tobacco use.[44,56] Coherence of the association implies that the epidemiological evidence should fit in well with the known biological and biochemical facts about the disease and the agent. This is clearly satisfied, as judged from clinical observation of the site of the cancer vs. habit relationship, that is, occurrence of cancer in locations that receive maximum exposure from tobacco use, and the diverse experimental findings demonstrating the carcinogenic potential of the constituents of tobacco. The criterion of specificity does not quite apply to tobacco and oral cancer because it is known that in addition to the oral cavity, tobacco causes cancers in various sites, and it also causes several other diseases. Also, it is well understood that cancer is an outcome of multiple factors.

Identification of tobacco (and TSNA) as the main agents for the causation of many cancers may stimulate research to prevent cancers by interventional and chemopreventive approaches. Modifications of tobacco products and agricultural practices to reduce the TSNA levels are also being attempted. Most important, however, is the fact that these epidemiological studies combined with experimental ones have advanced our understanding of the process of carcinogenesis, and perhaps will lead to a solution of the problem of cancer.

ACKNOWLEDGMENTS

This article was supported by Indo-U.S. Research Fund Agreement No. N-406-645. Dr. P. C. Gupta was supported by a Visiting Scientist Award at the International Agency for Research on Cancer, Lyon.

REFERENCES

1. **Parkin, D. M., Laara, E., and Muir, C. S.,** Estimates of the worldwide frequency of sixteen major cancers in 1980, *Int. J. Cancer,* 41, 184, 1988.

2. **U.S. Department of Health and Human Services,** Reducing the Health Consequences of Smoking, 25 Years of Progress, A Report of the Surgeon General, DHHS Publ. No. (CDC) 89-8411, U.S. Department of Health and Human Services, Public Health Service, 1989.

3. **World Health Organization,** Control of oral cancer in the developing countries, *Bull. WHO,* 62, 817, 1984.

4. **Parkin, D. M., Pisani, P., and Ferlay, J.,** Estimates of worldwide incidence of eighteen major cancers in 1985, *Int. J. Cancer,* 54, 594, 1993.

5. **Davis, S. and Severson, R. K.,** Increasing incidence of cancer of the tongue in the United States among young adults, *Lancet,* 2, 910, 1987.

6. **Coleman, M. P., Esteve, J., Damiecki, P., Arsian, A., and Renard, H.,** *Trends in Cancer Incidence and Mortality,* IARC Sci. Publ. No. 121, International Agency for Research on Cancer, Lyon.

7. **Pisani, P., Parkin, D. M., and Ferlay, J.,** Estimates of the worldwide mortality from eighteen major cancers in 1985: implications for prevention and projections of future burden, *Int. J. Cancer,* 55, 891, 1993.

8. **Indian Council of Medical Research,** National Cancer Registry Programme, Biennial Report 1988-89, New Delhi, 1992.

9. **International Agency for Research on Cancer,** *Tobacco Habits Other Than Smoking; Betel Quid and Areca-Nut Chewing; Some Related Nitrosamines,* Vol. 37, IARC Monographs on the Evaluation of Carcinogenic Risk of Chemicals to Humans, International Agency for Research on Cancer Sci. Publ., Lyon, 1985.

10. **International Agency for Research on Cancer,** *Tobacco Smoking,* IARC Monographs on the Evaluation of Carcinogenic Risk of Chemicals to Humans, Vol. 38, International Agency for Research on Cancer, Lyon, 1986.

11. **Pindborg, J. J., Murti, P. R., Bhonsle, R. B., and Gupta, P. C.,** Global aspects of tobacco use and its implications for oral health, in *Control of Tobacco-related Cancers and Other Diseases,* Gupta, P. C., Hamner, J. E., and Murti, P. R., Eds., Oxford University Press, Bombay, 1992, 13.

12. **Bhonsle, R. B., Murti, P. R., and Gupta, P. C.,** Tobacco habits in India, in *Control of Tobacco-related Cancers and Other Diseases,* Gupta, P. C., Hamner J. E., and Murti, P. R., Eds., Oxford University Press, Bombay, 1992, 26.

13. **Schoenborn, C. A. and Boyd, G.,** Smoking and other tobacco use: United States, 1987, National Center for Health Statistics, *Vital Health Stat.,* 10, 169, 1989.

14. **Sanghvi, L. D.,** Challenges in tobacco control in India: a historical perspective, in *Control of Tobacco-related Cancers and Other Diseases,* Gupta, P. C., Hamner, J. E., and Murti, P. R., Eds., Oxford University Press, Bombay, 1992, 47.

15. **WHO Database on Tobacco, India,** unpublished (personal communication).

16. **Hoffmann, D., Sanghvi, L. D., and Wynder, E. L.,** Chemical analysis of Indian *bidi* and American cigarette smoke, *Int. J. Cancer*, 14, 49, 1976.

17. **Hecht, S. S. and Hoffmann, D.,** Tobacco-specific nitrosamines, an important group of carcinogens in tobacco and tobacco smoke, *Carcinogenesis*, 9, 875, 1988.

18. **Hecht, S. S. and Hoffmann, D.,** The relevance of tobacco-specific nitrosamines to human cancer, *Cancer Surv.,* 8, 273, 1989.

19. **Bhide, S. V., Kulkami, J. R., Padma, P. R, Amonkar, A. J., Maru, G. B., Nair, U. J., and Nair, J.,** Studies on tobacco specific nitrosamines and other carcinogenic agents in smokeless tobacco products, in *Tobacco and Health, The Indian Scene*, Sanghvi, L. D. and Notani, P. N., Eds., Tata Memorial Centre, Bombay, 1989, 121.

20. **Hoffmann, D., Brunnemann, K. D., Hoffmann, I., Rivenson, A., and Hecht, S. S.,** Advances in tobacco carcinogenesis. II. Cigarette smoke, in *Control of Tobacco-related Cancers and Other Diseases*, Gupta, P. C., Hamner, J. E. and Murti, P. R., Eds., Oxford University Press, Bombay, 1992, 205.

21. **Hoffmann, D., Rivenson, A., Fung-Lung, C., and Hecht, H. H.,** Nicotine-derived N-nitrosamines (TSNA) and their relevance to tobacco carcinogenesis, *CRC Crit. Rev. Toxicol.*, 21, 305, 1991.

22. **Brunnemann, K. D. and Hoffmann, D.,** Chemical composition of smokeless tobacco products, in Smokeless Tobacco or Health, An International Perspective, NIH Publ. No. 92-3461, U.S. Department of Health and Human Services. Public Health Service, National Institutes of Health, 1992, 96.

23. **Redmond, D. E.,** Tobacco and cancer: the first clinical report, *N. Engl. J. Med.*, 282, 18, 1961.

24. **Abbey, R.,** Cancer of the mouth, the case against tobacco, *N.Y. Med. J.*, 102, 1, 1915.

25. **Niblock, W. J.,** Cancer in India, *Indian Med. Gaz.*, 37, 161, 1902.

26. **Fells, A.,** Cancel of the mouth in southern India, with an analysis of 209 operations, *Br. J. Cancer*, 2, 1357, 1902.

27. **Bentall, W. C.,** Cancer in Travancore, south India. A summary of 1700 cases, *Br. Med. J.*, 2, 1428, 1908.

28. **Orr, I. M.,** Oral cancer in betel-nut chewers in Travancore: its aetiology, pathology and treatment, *Lancet*, 2, 575, 1933.

29. **Gupta, P. C., Pindborg, J. J., and Mehta, F. S.,** Comparison of carcinogenecity of betel quid with and without tobacco, an epidemiological review, *Ecol. Dis.*, 1, 213, 1982.

30. **U.S. Department of Health and Human Services,** The Health Consequences of Smoking, Cancer, DHHS Publ. No. (OHS) 82-50179, 1982.

31. **U.S. Department of Health and Human Services,** Health Implications of Smokeless Tobacco Use, National Institutes of Health Consensus Development Conference (Vol. 6, No. 1), U.S. Department of Health and Human Services, Public Health Service, National Institutes of Health, Office of Medical Applications of Research, 1986.

32. **U.S. Department of Health and Human Services,** Health Consequences of Using Smokeless Tobacco, A Report of the Advisory Committee to the Surgeon General, NIH Publ. No. 86-2874, U.S. Department of Health and Human Services, Public Health Service, National Institutes of Health, 1986.

33. **Parkin, D. M., Muir, C. S., Whelan, S. L., Gao, Y. T., Ferlay J., and Powell, J.,** Cancer Incidence in Five Continents, Vol. VI, IARC Sci. Publ. No. 120. International Agency for Research on Cancer, Lyon, 1992.

34. **Franco, E. L., Kowaiski, L. P., Oliveira, B. V., Curado, M. P., Pereira, R. N., Silver, M. E., Fava, A. S., and Torloni, H.,** Risk factors for oral cancer in Brazil: a case-control study, *Int. J. Cancer*, 43, 992, 1989.

35. **Oreggia, F., Stefani, E. D., Correa, P., and Fierro, l.,** Risk factors for cancer of the tongue in Uruguay, *Cancer*, 67, 180, 1991.

36. **Merletti, F., Boffetta, P., Ciccone, G., Mashberg, A., and Terracini, B.,** Role of tobacco and alcoholic beverages in the etiology of cancer of the oral cavity\oropharynx in Torino, Italy, **Cancer Res.**, 49, 4919, 1989.

37. **Negri, E., La-Vecchia, C., Franceschi, S., and Tavani, A.,** Attributable risk for oral

cancer in northern Italy, *Cancer Epidemiol. Biomarkers Prev.*, 2, 189, 1993.

38. **Wahi, P. N.,** The epidemiology of oral and oro-pharyngeal cancer. A report of the study in Mainpuri District, Uttar Pradesh, India, *Bull. WHO*, 38, 495, 1961.

39. **Hirayama, T.,** An epidemiological study of oral and pharyngeal cancer in Central and Southeast Asia, *Bull. WHO*, 34, 41, 1966.

40. **Jussawalla, D. J. and Deshpande, V. A.,** Evaluation of cancer risk in tobacco chewers and smokers: an epidemiologic assessment, *Cancer*, 28, 244, 1971.

41. **Jafarey, N. A., Mehmood, Z., and Zaidi, S. H. M.,** Habits and dietary patterns of cases of carcinoma of the oral cavity and oropharynx, *J. Pak. Med. Assoc.*, 27, 340, 1977.

42. **Sankaranarayanan, R., Duffy, S. W., Day, N. E., Nair, M. K., and Padmakumary, G.,** A case-control investigation of cancer of the oral tongue and the floor of the mouth in southern India, *Int. J. Cancer*, 4, 617, 1989.

43. **Nandakumar, A., Thimmasetty, K. T., Sreeramareddy, N. Mh., Venugopal, T. C., Rajanna, Vinutha, A. T., Srinivas, and Bhargava, M. K.,** A population based case-control investigation on cancers of the oral cavity in Bangalore, India, *Br. J. Cancer*, 62, 847, 1990.

44. **Bhargava, K., Smith, L. W., Mani, N. J., Silverman, S., Jr., Malaowalla, A. M., and Billimoria, K. F.,** A follow-up study of oral cancer and precancerous lesions in 57,518 industrial workers of Gujarat, India, *Indian J. Cancer*, 12, 124, 1975.

45. **Sanghvi, L. D., Rao, K. C. M., and Khanolkar, V. R.,** Smoking and chewing of tobacco in relation to cancer of the upper alimentary tract, *Br. Med. J.*, 1, 1111, 1955.

46. **Sanghvi, L. D., Jayant, K., and Pakhale, S. S.,** Tobacco use and cancer in India, *World Smoking and Health*, 5, 4, 1980.

47. **Jussawalla, D. J.,** Different types of smoking and chewing habits in India, in *The UICC Smoking Control Workshop*, Tominaga, S. and Aoki, K., Eds., University of Nagoya Press, Nagoya, 1982, 40.

48. **Jayant, K. and Pakhale, S. S.,** Toxic constituents in *bidi* smoke, in *Tobacco or Health, The Indian Scene*, Sanghvi, L. D. and Notani, P. N., Eds., Tata Memorial Centre, Bombay, 1989, 101.

49. **Bhide, S.,** Carcinogenic potential of some Indian tobacco products, in *Control of Tobacco-Related Cancers and Other Diseases*, Gupta, P. C., Hamner, J. E., and Murti, P. R., Eds., Oxford University Press, Bombay, 1992, 217.

50. **Reddy, D. G. and Rao, V. K.,** Cancer of the palate in coastal Andhra due to smoking cigars with the burning end inside the mouth, *Indian J. Med. Sci.*, 11, 791, 1957.

51. **Reddy, C. R. R. R. M. and Ramulu, C.,** Review of carcinoma of hard palate in Visakhapatnam area and its etiopathogenesis, *Clinician*, 36, 131, 1972.

52. **Khanolkar, V. R. and Suryabai, B.,** Cancer in relation to usages. Three new types in India, *Arch. Pathol.*, 40, 351, 1945.

53. **Khanolkar, V. R.,** Oral cancer in India, *Acta Unio Int. Contra Cancrum*, 15, 67, 1959.

54. **Shanta, V. and Krishnamurthy, S.,** A study of aetiological factors in oral squamous cell carcinoma, *Br. J. Cancer*, 13, 382, 1959.

55. **Wahi, P. N., Lahiri, B., Kehar, U., and Arora, S.,** Oral and oro-pharyngeal cancer in North India, *Br. J. Cancer*, 19, 627, 1965.

56. **Gupta, P. C., Mehta, F. S., Daftary, D. K., Pindborg, J. J., Bhonsle, R. B., Jalnawalla, P. N., Sinor, P. N., Pitkar, V. K., Murti, P. R., Irani, R. R., Shah, H. T., Kadam, P. M., Iyer, K. S. S., Iyer, H. M., Hegde, A. K., Chandrasekhar, G. K., Shroff, B. C., Sahiar, B. E., and Mehta, M. M.,** Incidence rates of oral cancer and natural history of oral precancerous lesions in a 10-year follow-up study of Indian villagers, *Community Dent. Oral Epidemiol.*, 8, 287, 1980.

57. **Reddy, D. G., Reddy, D. B., and Rao, P. R.,** Experimental production of cancer with tobacco tar and heat, *Cancer*, 13, 263, 1960.

58. **Vogler, W. R., Lloyd, J. W., and Milmore, B. K.,** A retrospective study of etiological factors in cancer of the mouth, pharynx, and larynx, *Science*, 15, 246, 1962.

59. **Vincent, R. G. and Marchetta, F.,** The relationship of the use of tobacco and alcohol to cancer of the oral cavity, pharynx, or larynx, *Am. J. Surg.*, 106, 501, 1963.

60. **Martinez, I.,** Factors associated with cancer of the esophagus, mouth, and pharynx in Puerto Rico, *J. Natl. Cancer Inst.*, 42, 1069, 1969.

61. **Win, D. M., Blot, W. J., Shy, C. M., Pickle, C. W., Toledo, A., and Fraumeni, J. F., Jr.,** Snuff dipping and oral cancer among women in the southern United States, *N. Engl. J. Med.*, 304, 745, 1981.

62. **Winn, D. M.,** Surveillance of and knowledge about cancer associated with smokeless tobacco use, in Smokeless Tobacco or Health, An International perspective, NIH Publ. No. 92-3461, U.S. Department of Health and Human Services, Public Health Service, National Institutes of Health, 1992, 11.

63. **Hoffmann, D., Rivenson, A., Prokopczyk, B., Brunnemann, K. D., Carmella, S. G., and Hoffmann, I.,** Advances in tobacco carcinogenesis. I. Smokeless tobacco and betel quid, in *Control of Tobacco-Related Cancers and Other Diseases*, Gupta, P. C., Hamner, J. E., and Murti, P. R., Eds., Oxford University Press, Bombay, 1992, 193.

64. **Paymaster, J. C. and Gangadharan, P.,** Cancer in the Parsi community of Bombay, *Int. J. Cancer*, 5, 426, 1970.

65. **Ahluwalia, H. S., Duguid, J. B.,** Malignant tumors in Malaya, *Br. J. Cancer*, 20, 12, 1966.

66. **Paymaster, J. C.,** Some observations on oral and pharyngeal cancer carcinomas in the state of Bombay, *Cancer*, 15, 578, 1962.

67. **Simarak, S., de Jong, U. W., Breslow, N., Dahl, C. W., Ruckphaopunt, K., Scheelings, P., and Maclennan, R.,** Cancer of the oral cavity, pharynx/larynx, and lung in northern Thailand, case-control study and analysis of cigar smoke, *Br. J. Cancer*, 36, 130, 1977.

68. **Sankaranarayanan, R., Duffy, S. W., Padmakumary, G., Day, N. E., and Padmanabhan, T. K.,** Tobacco chewing, alcohol and snuff in cancer of gingiva in Kerala, India, *Br. J. Cancer*, 60, 638, 1989.

69. **Sankaranarayanan, R., Duffy, S. W., Padmakumary, G., Day, N. E., and Nair, M. K.,** Risk factors for cancers of the buccal and labial mucosa in Kerala, South India, *J. Epidemiol. Community Health*, 44, 286, 1990.

70. **Mehta, F. S., Pindborg, J. J., Gupta, P. C., and Daftary, D. K.,** Epidemiologic and histologic study of oral cancer and leukoplakia among 50,915 villagers in India, *Cancer*, 24, 832, 1969.

71. **Mehta, F. S., Gupta, P. C., Daftary, D. K., Pindborg, J. J., and Choksi, S. K.,** An epidemiologic study of oral cancer and precancerous conditions among 101,761 villagers in Maharashtra, *Int. J. Cancer*, 10, 134, 1972.

72. **Mehta, F. S., Aghi, M. B., Gupta, P. C., Pindborg, J. J., Bhonsle, R. B., Jalnawalla, P. N., and Sinor, P. N.,** An intervention study of oral cancer and precancer in rural Indian populations, a preliminary report, *Bull. WHO*, 60, 441, 1982.

73. **Gupta, P. C., Mehta, F. S., Pindborg, J. J., Bhonsle, R. B., Daftary, D. K., Murti, P. R., and Shah, H. T.,** Intervention study for primary prevention of oral cancer among 36,000 Indian tobacco users, *Lancet*, 1, 1235, 1986.

74. **Gupta, P. C., Mehta, F. S., Pindborg, J. J., Bhonsle, R. B., Murti, P. R., Daftary, D. K., and Aghi, M. B.,** Primary prevention trial on oral cancer in India: a 10-year follow-up study, *J. Oral Pathol. Med.*, 21, 433, 1992.

75. **Gupta, P. C., Bhonsle, R. B., Murti, P. R., Daftary, D. K., Mehta, F. S., and Pindborg, J.,** An epidemiologic assessment of cancer risk in oral precancerous lesions

in India with special reference to nodular leukoplakia, *Cancer*, 63, 2247, 1989.

76. **Van Wyk, C. W., Stander, I., Padayachee, A., and Grobler-Rabie, A. F.,** The areca nut chewing habit and oral squamous cell carcinoma in South African Indians, a retrospective study, *S. Afr. Med. J.*, 83, 425, 1993.

77. **Wahi, P. N., Kehar, U., and Lahiri, B.,** Factors influencing oral and oro-pharyngeal cancers in India, *Br. J. Cancer*, 19, 642, 1965.

78. **Nugmanov, S. N. and Bainakanov, S. S.,** The result of an epidemiological study of orpharyngeal tumors in Kazakhstan following the WHO Project, in *Epidemiology of Malignant Tumors*, Nauka, Alma-Ata, 1970, 227.

79. **Ibrahim, E. M., Satti, M. B., Al-Idrissi, H. Y., Higazi, M. M., Magbool, G. M., and Al-Quorain, A.,** Oral cancer in Saudi Arabia, the role of alqat and alshamma, *Cancer Detect. Prev.*, 9, 215, 1986.

80. **Soufi, H. E., Kameswaran, M., and Maltani, T.,** Khat and oral cancer, *J. Laryngol. Otol.*, 105, 643, 1991.

81. **Hanan, M. A., el-Yazigi, A., Paul, M., Gibson, D. P., and Philips, R. L.,** Genotoxicity of shamma, a chewing material suspected of causing oral cancer in Saudi Arabia, *Mutat. Res.*, 169, 41, 1986.

Critical Reviews in Toxicology, 26(2):199–211 (1996)

The Biological Significance of Tobacco-Specific *N*-Nitrosamines: Smoking and Adenocarcinoma of the Lung

Dietrich Hoffmann, Abraham Rivenson, and Stephen S. Hecht
Naylor Dana Institute for Disease Prevention, American Health Foundation, Valhalla, NY 10595

ABSTRACT: In the U.S., there has been a steeper rise of the incidence of lung adenocarcinoma than of squamous cell carcinoma of the lung among cigarette smokers. Since 1950, the percentage of all cigarettes sold that had filter tips increased from 0.56 to 92% in 1980 and to 97% in 1990. The tobacco of the filter cigarettes is richer in nitrate than that of the nonfilter cigarettes manufactured in past decades. Because the smoker of cigarettes with lower nicotine yield tends to smoke more intensely and to inhale the smoke more deeply than the smoker of plain cigarettes, the peripheral lung is exposed to higher amounts of nitrogen oxides, nitrosated compounds, and lung-specific smoke carcinogens. It is our working hypothesis that more intense smoking, deeper inhalation of the smoke, and higher smoke delivery of the organ-specific lung carcinogen NNK to the peripheral lung are major contributors to the increased risk of cigarette smokers for lung adenocarcinoma. Bioassay data and biochemical studies in support of this concept are discussed.

KEY WORDS: tobacco-specific *N*-nitrosamines (TSNA), lung adenocarcinoma (AC), 4-(methyl-nitrosamino)-1-(3-pyridyl)-1-butanone (NNK), metabolic activation, K-*ras* oncogene activation, SCC, squamous cell carcinoma.

I. INTRODUCTION

In 1990, at the 15th International Cancer Congress in Hamburg, Germany, a "Round Table Discussion" was held on tobacco-specific *N*-nitrosamines (TSNA).[1] As reflected in the preceding papers of this Symposium, remarkable progress has been made in the chemistry, biochemistry, and molecular biology related to TSNA and in the epidemiology of tobacco-associated cancer. TSNA are known to induce benign and malignant tumors of the lung, oral cavity, esophagus, pancreas, and liver.

This overview focuses on the biological significance of TSNA and on our current understanding of their contribution to the induction of lung cancer in cigarette smokers.

It is well established that tobacco chewing and especially snuff dipping are causally associated with cancer of the oral cavity, while tobacco smoking is a cause of cancer of the lung and cancer of the upper aerodigestive tract, pancreas, renal pelvis, and urinary bladder.[2–5] Tobacco contains more than 3000 compounds, including 30 carcinogens, and tobacco smoke has more than 4000 constituents, including about 50 carcinogens.[6–8] It appears to be an insurmountable task to delineate the contribution of single groups of agents, such as TSNA, to the induction of cancer at specific sites. We review the epidemiological and experimental data that have accrued in support of the concept that TSNA, and especially 4-(methylnitrosamino)-1-(3-pyridyl)-1-

butanone (NNK) and its reduction product 4-(methylnitrosamino)-1-(3-pyridyl)-1-butanol (NNAL), are important causal factors for the association of cigarette smoking with adenocarcinoma of the lung.

II. ADENOCARCINOMA OF THE LUNG — EPIDEMIOLOGICAL STUDIES

The first large-scale study in the U.S. in 1950 reported that 597 of 605 male lung cancer cases had a history of cigarette smoking and that among these, 35 had adenocarcinoma (AC); the remaining cases were classified as squamous cell carcinoma (SCC). The ratio of AC to SCC was 1:16;[9] however, among 728 new male lung cancer cases between 1970 and 1976, the ratio had changed to 1:2.24,[10] and among 1278 lung cancer cases examined in the years 1977 to 1984, to 1:1.58.[11] Between 1964 and 1971, the Baptist Memorial Hospital in Memphis, TN, char-

acterized 868 male lung cancer cases and found the ratio of AC to SCC to be 1:3.1; between 1972 and 1978 among 1388 male lung cancer cases, the ratio was 1:2.9, and between 1979 and 1985, among 1483 male lung cancer cases, the AC:SCC ratio was 1:1.6.[12] Several additional hospital-based studies in the U.S.[13–15] and population-based studies[16–19] confirmed the observation that the ratio of AC to SCC in male lung cancer cases has gradually changed toward AC. Table 1 presents analyses done at the National Cancer Institute for a segment comprising about 7% of the U.S. population for the periods 1969–1971 and 1984 to 1986.[19] In this comparison, the ratio of AC to SCC among male lung cancer cases changed from 1:2.4 to 1:1.4 and, just as importantly, in these periods the incidence rates among white males increased for SCC by 25% and for AC by 111%; the incidence rates among black males increased by 50 and 151%, respectively.[19] Clearly, these studies document a change in the ratio of the two major types of

TABLE 1
Lung Cancer Trends by Histologic Type from Five Geographic Areas of the U.S., 1969–1971 and 1984–1986

	1969–1971		1984–1986		% Change
	No.	Rate[a]	No.	Rate[a]	
White males					
Squamous cell carcinoma	3767	21.7	5100	27.2	25
Adenocarcinoma	1638	9.3	3685	19.6	111
Black males					
Squamous cell carcinoma	543	33.8	1070	50.6	50
Adenocarcinoma	193	11.5	633	28.9	151
White females					
Squamous cell carcinoma	566	2.7	1658	6.9	156
Adenocarcinoma	747	3.5	2572	11.2	220
Black females					
Squamous cell carcinoma	67	3.4	291	10.5	209
Adenocarcinoma	75	3.8	340	12.2	221

a Rate per 100,000 person-years, directly age adjusted using the 1970 U.S. standard.

From Devesa, S. S., Shaw, G. L., and Blot, W. J., *Cancer Epidemiol. Biomarkers Prev.*, 1, 29, 1991. With permission.

lung cancer in men, and, more significantly, they show a steeper increase in the incidence rates of adenocarcinoma compared with squamous cell carcinoma. In 1991, an estimated 90.3% of the 92,000 deaths from lung cancer in men and 78.5% of the 51,000 lung cancer deaths in women in the U.S. were attributable to cigarette smoking.[20]

On the basis of epidemiological studies, one would assume that an increase in lung cancer incidence, in general, and a more rapid increase of one histological type of lung cancer would be primarily associated with the consumption of cigarettes, although other factors or cofactors, such as concurrent exposure to asbestos or polonium-210, may play a role in the increase of SCC and AC in the lung.

III. THE CHANGING CIGARETTE

During the past 4 decades, the sales-weighted average smoke yields of American cigarettes have declined from 38 mg of "tar" and 2.7 mg of nicotine per cigarette to 13.5 and 0.9 mg, respectively (Figure 1).[21] These "tar" and nicotine yields resulted from stan-

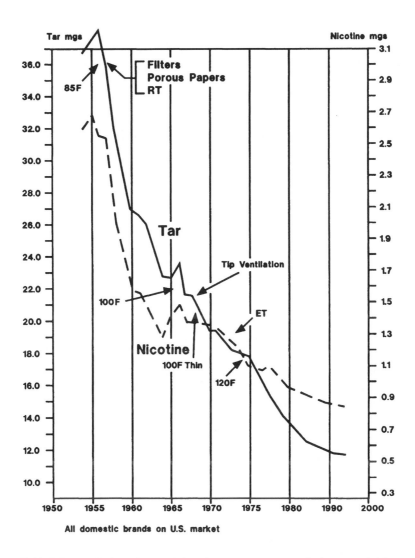

FIGURE 1. U.S. sales-weighted average "tar" and nicotine yields, 1954–1993. RT, reconstituted tobacco; F, filter; ET, expanded tobacco.

dardized machine-smoking conditions that were based on observations of smokers in 1936.[22] The conditions are one puff per minute, with a puff duration of 2 s and a puff volume of 35 ml. These standards were accepted by the U.S. Federal Trade Commission in 1969 for comparing the relative smoke yields of all brands of commercial cigarettes.[23] Whereas these conditions may reflect the smoking habits of a smoker of a high-yield cigarette, they do not apply to the majority of the U.S. smokers of low-yield filter cigarettes. In 1950, 0.56% of the cigarettes smoked in America had filter tips. Since that time, the market share of filter-tipped cigarettes increased gradually to 51% in 1960, 80% in 1970, 92% in 1980, and to more than 97% in 1992.[21] Clearly, the determining factor for the smoking intensity is the smoker's dependence on nicotine.[24] To satisfy a craving for nicotine, a smoker of low-yield filter cigarettes may take up to five puffs per minute with volumes up to 55 ml, while the duration of drawing a puff remains close to 2 s. In addition, more than 50% of present-day filter cigarettes have perforated filter tips, which allow dilution of the smoke generated during puffing with air that enters the smoke stream through the holes in the filter. Intentionally or unintentionally, the smoker of these cigarettes may close the holes with fingers and/or lips and thereby negate, to various extents, the intended effect of the smoke dilution by air. Furthermore, the velocity of the smoke drawn through the burning cone and tobacco column is higher.[25–29] When a smoking machine is programmed to simulate the smoking characteristics of a filter cigarette smoker, the smoke yields increase two- to threefold for "tar", nicotine, and carbon monoxide, and also for most known tobacco smoke carcinogens such as benzo(a)pyrene (BaP) and TSNA.[30–32] Most smokers of low-nicotine cigarettes appear to inhale smoke more deeply than do the smokers of nonfilter cigarettes.[33] As a result of more intense smoking and deeper inhalation of the smoke, the bronchioalveolar regions

and the smaller bronchi of the smoker are exposed to disproportionately higher amounts of "tar" and carcinogenic agents such as certain volatile aldehydes, polynuclear aromatic hydrocarbons (PAH), aromatic amines, and volatile and tobacco-specific N-nitrosamines. Unlike the bronchi, the bronchioles have limited defense mechanisms. The concept that deeper inhalation may cause primarily AC in the distant lung is supported by data showing that most neoplasms among primary smokers of cigars and pipes — who do not inhale smoke deeply — are SCC arising from the major bronchi.[5]

The epidemiology of smoking and lung cancer, and observations on the changing smoking patterns of consumers of low-yield filter cigarettes, have led to development of a working hypothesis that supports the observation of an increased risk for lung AC in cigarette smokers. The factors of major significance are (1) the organ specificity of the carcinogenic TSNA, especially that of NNK, and (2) the more intense smoking and deeper inhalation of the smoke of filter cigarettes due to their low nicotine content.

IV. CARCINOGENICITY OF TSNA

Several N-nitrosamines are organ-specific procarcinogens that require metabolic activation to reactive species in specific target organs independent of the mode of application. In the case of TSNA, 4-(methylnitrosamino)-1-(3-pyridyl)-1-butanone (NNK), and its reduction product 4-(methylnitrosamino)-1-(3-pyridyl)-1-butanol (NNAL), two powerful carcinogens, the major target organ is the lung, especially the peripheral part of the lung.[34,35] This occurs independent of the route of administration, whether these procarcinogens are applied topically to the skin, taken orally, or by intraperitoneal, subcutaneous or intravesical injection. The tumors induced by these TSNA are adenoma and AC of the lung (Table 2).[36–52] The metabolic activation

TABLE 2
Carcinogenicity of NNK and NNAL in Laboratory Animals

Animal	Strain	Route or application	Target organs	Dose (mmol/animal)	Ref.
NNK					
Mouse	Sencar	Topical (TI)[a]	Lung, skin	0.0014–0.028	36
	A/J	Intraperitoneal	Lung	0.0025–0.01	37
	A/J	Intraperitoneal	Lung	0.005–0.02	38
	A/J	Intraperitoneal	Lung	0.008–0.024	39
	A/J	Intragastric	Lung	0.008–0.024	39
	NIH-Swiss newborn	Intraperitoneal	Lung, liver	0.0004	40
Rat	F344	Oral-swabbing	Lung, nasal cavity	2.6	41
		Oral-gavage	Lung, liver	1.3	42
		Oral-drinking water	Lung, pancreas, liver	0.075–0.31	43
		Subcutaneous	Lung, nasal cavity, liver	3.4	44
		Subcutaneous	Lung, nasal cavity, liver	0.17–2.5	45
		Subcutaneous	Lung, nasal cavity, liver	0.009–2.8	46
		Intravesicular	Lung, liver	1.5	47
Hamster	Syrian golden	Subcutaneous	Lung, nasal cavity	0.91	48
		Subcutaneous	Lung	0.05	49
		Subcatenous	Lung	~0.6	50
		Subcatenous	Lung	~0.5	51
NNAL					
Mouse	A/J	Intraperitoneal	Lung	0.005–0.101	52
	A/J	Intraperitoneal	Lung	0.01–0.05	38

[a] TI, tumor initiator (ten subdoses) followed by 40 TPA applications (total dose 80 mg of TPA).

occurs in the Clara cells and other cell types of the lung.[46]

The most abundant carcinogenic TSNA in tobacco and mainstream smoke is N'-nitrosonornicotine (NNN).[35] It induces in mice primarily lung tumors, in rats tumors of the esophagus and nasal cavity, in Syrian golden hamsters tumors of the trachea and nasal cavity, and in minks tumors of the nasal cavity. N'-Nitrosoanabasine (NAB) is a weak carcinogen whose major target organ is the lung in mice and the esophagus in rats, whereas the other three identified TSNA — N'-nitrosoanatabine (NAT), 4-(methylnitrosamino)-4-(3-pyridyl)-1-butanol (iso-NNAL), and 4-(methylnitrosamino)-4-(3-pyridyl) butyric acid (iso-NNAC) — are most likely not carcinogenic (Table 3).[36,38,44,45,48,52–64]

Up to 180 ng per cigarette of the major organ-specific lung carcinogen NNK are found in the mainstream smoke (MS) of a cigarette when smoked under standardized laboratory conditions, and up to 130 ng are generated in the MS from a low-yield filter cigarette smoked under intensive smoking conditions such as observed in filter smokers.[31,65] Assuming that a smoker (70 kg) consumes 40 nonfilter cigarettes per day for 40 years, this translates into a respiratory tract exposure to about 1.4 mg/kg and for a smoker of a filter cigarette up to 1.0 mg/kg of the carcinogen, respectively. The lowest dose required to induce lung adenoma in rats is 0.03 mg/kg administered three times weekly for 20 weeks for a total of 1.8 mg/kg.[46] Clearly, these data support the concept that NNK in cigarette smoke represents a risk

TABLE 3

Carcinogenicity of NNN, NAB, NAT, *Iso*-NNAL and *Iso*-NNAC

Animal/ strain	Route of administration	Target organs	Dose (mmol/animal)	Ref.
		NNN		
eMouse				
Sencar	Topical (TI)[a]	None	0.028	36
Chester Beatty	Intraperitoneal	Lung	0.46	53
A/J	Intraperitoneal	Lung	0.12	52
	Intraperitoneal	Lung	0.02–0.1	38
Rat				
F344	Oral, drinking water	Esophagus, nasal cavity	3.6	54
	Oral, drinking water	Esophagus, nasal cavity	3.3–3.6	55
Sprague Dawley	Oral, drinking water	Nasal cavity	9.3	56
F344	Oral, drinking water	Esophagus, nasal cavity, tongue	1.0	57
BDV1	Oral, gavage	Nasal cavity	0.26–2.6	58
F344	Subcutaneous	Nasal cavity	3.4	44
	Subcutaneous	Nasal cavity, esophagus, lung	0.17–2.6	45
	Subcutaneous	nasal cavity	1.0	54
Hamster				
Syrian golden	Subcutaneous	Trachea	2.1	59
	Subcutaneous	Trachea	0.91	48
	Intraperitoneal	Trachea, nasal cavity	1.0–2.0	60
	Oral, drinking water	Trachea, nasal cavity	1.9–2.8	55
Mink	Subcutaneous	Nasal cavity	11.9	61
		NAB		
Mouse				
A/J	Intraperitoneal	Lung	0.1	38
Rat				
Chester Beatty	Oral, drinking water	Esophagus	7.7	62
F344	Oral, drinking water	Esophagus	3.3	54
Hamster				
Syrian golden	Subcutaneous	None	2.0	59
		NAT		
Rat				
F344	Subcutaneous	None	0.16–2.5	45
		***Iso*-NNAL**		
Mouse				
Sencar	Topical (TI)[a]	None	0.059	36
C57BL	Oral gavage	None	1.0	63
A/J	Intraperitoneal	None	0.2	38
Rat				
F344	Oral, drinking water	None	4.0	63
		***Iso*-NNAC**		
Mouse				
A/J	Intraperitoneal	None	0.2	64
	Intraperitoneal	None	0.2	38

[a] TI, tumor initiator (ten subdoses) followed by 40 TPA applications (total dose, 80 µg of TPA).

factor for the induction of lung adeno-carcinoma in long-term cigarette smokers.

V. BIOCHEMISTRY OF TSNA

It is well established that the carcino-genic TSNA are metabolically activated by α-hydroxylation.[66] In the case of the strong lung carcinogen NNK, the metabolic activation in rat lung occurs by oxidative enzyme systems in the Clara cells and in other cell types. The hydroxylation of the methyl group of NNK leads to the unstable 4-oxo-4-(3-pyridyl)butane diazohydroxide, which forms pyridyloxobutylated DNA (Figure 2).[66] After acid treatment, this DNA adduct releases 4-hydroxy-1-(3-pyridyl)-1-butanone (HPB). The α-hydroxylation of the methylene group of NNK leads to the unstable 4-hydroxy-4-(methylnitrosamino)-1-(3-pyridyl)-1-butanone, which decomposes to 4-oxo-4-

(3-pyridyl)butanal and methane diazo-hydroxide. The latter reacts with DNA to form methylated bases, including O^6-methyl-guanine (O^6mG) and 7-methylguanine. O^6mG has been quantified in the lung DNA of rats and mice.[67,68] The formation of these DNA adducts has been correlated with the expression of point mutations in the K-ras gene in mice, and is considered to be an important event in the cascade of cellular changes leading to the development of NNK-induced ACs of the lung.[69]

In the human lung, levels of 7-methyl-guanine formed by NNK, and possibly by other methylating species in tobacco smoke, are higher in cigarette smokers than in non-smokers.[70] Levels of DNA-pyridyloxy-butylation are also higher in the lung and trachea of smokers than of nonsmokers.[71]

Twenty to 30% of cigarette smokers with AC were found to have activated K-ras genes with mutations in codon 12 in their lung

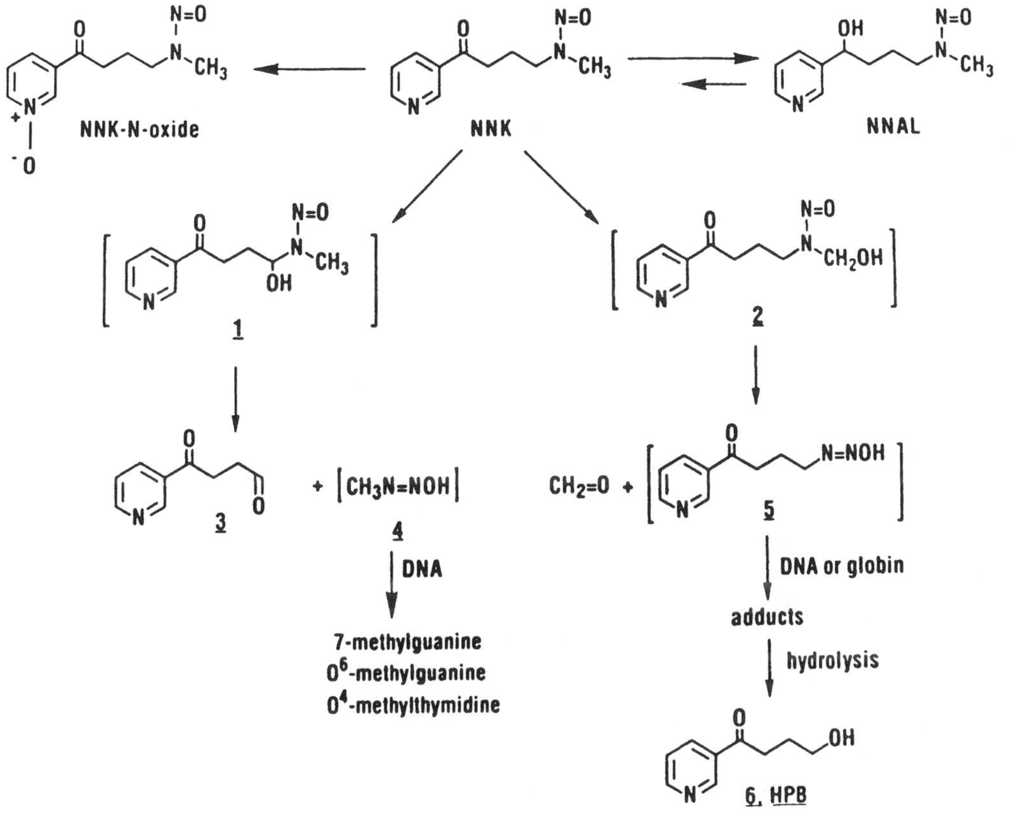

FIGURE 2. Overview of metabolism of NNK by α-hydroxylation.[65]

tissues.[72,73] These mutations are defined as approximately 80% guanine-thymine (G-T) transversions and 20% guanine-adenine (G-A) transitions.[72] In A/J mice and in Syrian golden hamsters, AC induced by NNK contain activated K-ras genes, with mostly G-A transitions in codon 12.[51,74] In the rat, activated K-ras genes have so far not been detected in lung tumors.[74] Comparison of activated K-ras genes in lung tumors induced by methylating and pyridyloxybutylating agents in the A/J mouse have demonstrated that the methylating agent causes G-A transitions on codon 12, whereas the pyridyloxobutylating agent induces both G-A transitions and G-T transversions.[75] Thus, it appears that the G-T transversions in codon 12 of the K-ras gene observed in lung AC of cigarette smokers could result from the NNK or NNN pyridyloxobutylation pathway, as well as from other tobacco smoke carcinogens such as PAH, volatile aldehydes, nitroalkanes, and other agents.

These data support the observation that cigarette smoking causes lung AC. They are consistent with our working hypothesis that the increase in NNK and a decrease of BaP[76] in the smoke of cigarettes with low-nicotine delivery plays a role in the more pronounced increase of AC over SCC in the lungs of cigarette smokers.

VI. SUMMARY

In the U.S., there has been a steeper rise of the incidence of lung adenocarcinoma than of squamous cell carcinoma of the lung among cigarette smokers. Since 1950, the percentage of all cigarettes sold that had filter tips increased from 0.56 to 92% in 1980, to 97% in 1990. The tobacco of the filter cigarettes is richer in nitrate than that of the nonfilter cigarettes manufactured in past decades. Because the smoker of cigarettes with lower nicotine yield tends to smoke more intensely and to inhale the smoke more deeply than the smoker of plain ciga-

rettes, the peripheral lung is exposed to higher amounts of nitrogen oxides, nitrosated compounds, and lung-specific smoke carcinogens. It is our working hypothesis that more intense smoking, deeper inhalation of the smoke, and higher smoke delivery of the organ-specific lung carcinogen NNK to the peripheral lung are major contributors to the increased risk of cigarette smokers for lung adenocarcinoma. Bioassay data and biochemical studies in support of this concept are discussed.

ACKNOWLEDGMENTS

We appreciate the editorial assistance of Ilse Hoffmann and Jennifer Johnting. Our studies are supported by Grants No. CA-29850 and CA-44377 and by the Cancer Center Grant No. CA-17613 from the National Cancer Institute.

REFERENCES

1. **Hoffmann, D. and Spiegelhalder, B.,** Eds., Tobacco-specific nitrosamines. Round table discussion, 15th International Cancer Congress, August 1990, Hamburg, Germany, *Crit. Rev. Toxicol.*, 21, 235, 1991.

2. **International Agency for Research on Cancer,** Tobacco Habits Other than Smoking; Betel Quid and Areca-Nut Chewing; and some Related Nitrosamines, IARC Monograph on the Evaluation of the Carcinogenic Risk of Chemicals to Humans, Lyon, 37, 1985.

3. **United States Surgeon General,** The Health Consequences of Using Smokeless Tobacco, NIH Publ. No. 86-2874, 1986.

4. **International Agency for Research on Cancer,** Tobacco Smoking. IARC Monograph on the Evaluation of the Carcinogenic Risk of Chemicals to Humans, Lyon, 1986, 38.

5. **U.S. Surgeon General,** Reducing the Health Consequences of Smoking. 25 Years of

Progress, DHHS Publ. No. (CDC)89-8411, 1989.

6. **Roberts, N. L.,** Natural tobacco flavor, *Recent Adv. Tob. Sci.,* 14, 49, 1988.

7. **Brunnemann, K. D. and Hoffmann, D.,** Chemical Composition of Tobacco Products, National Cancer Institute Smoking, Tobacco Control Monograph 2, Smokeless Tobacco and Health, NIH Publ. No. 93-3461, 1993.

8. **Hoffmann, D. and Hoffmann, I.,** Tobacco consumption and lung cancer, in *Lung Cancer. Advances in Basic and Clinical Research,* H. H. Hansen, Ed., Kluwer, Boston, 1994, 1–42.

9. **Wynder, E. L. and Graham, E. G.,** Tobacco smoking as a possible etiologic factor in bronchiogenic carcinoma, *J. Am. Med. Assoc.,* 143, 329, 1950.

10. **Wynder, E. L. and Stellman, S. D.,** Comparative epidemiology of tobacco-related cancers, *Cancer Res.,* 37, 4608, 1977.

11. **Wynder, E. L. and Covey, L. S.,** Epidemiologic patterns in lung cancer by histologic type, *Eur. J. Cancer Clin. Oncol.,* 23, 1491, 1987.

12. **El-Torky, M., El-Zeky, F., and Hall, J. C.,** Significant changes in the distribution of histologic type of lung cancer. A review of 4,928 cases, *Cancer,* 65, 1647, 1990.

13. **Vincent, R. G., Pickren, J. W., Lane, W. W., Bross, I., Takita, H., Honten, L., Guierrez, A. C., and Rzepka, T.,** The changing histopathology of lung cancer, *Cancer,* 39, 1647, 1977.

14. **Cox, J. D. and Yesner, R. A.,** Adenocarcinoma of the lung: recent results from the Veterans Administration lung group, *Am. Rev. Respir. Dis.,* 120, 1025, 1979.

15. **Johnston, W. W.,** Histologic and cytologic patterns of lung cancer in 2,580 men and women over a 15-year period, *Acta. Cytol.,* 32, 163, 1988.

16. **Cutler, S. J. and Young, J. L.,** Third National Cancer Survey: incidence data, *J. Natl. Cancer Inst. Monogr.,* 41, 1, 1975.

17. **Young, J. L., Percy, C. L., and Asire, A. J., Eds.,** Cancer incidence and mortality in the United States, 1973–1977, *J. Natl. Cancer Inst. Monogr.,* 57, 1, 1981.

18. **Beard, M. C., Annegers, J. F., Woolner, L. B., and Kurland, L. T.,** Bronchiogenic carcinoma in Olmsted County, 1935–1979, *Cancer,* 55, 2026, 1985.

19. **Devesa, S. S., Shaw, G. L., and Blot, W. J.,** Changing patterns of lung cancer incidence by histologic type, *Cancer Epidemiol. Biomarkers Prev.,* 1, 29, 1991.

20. **Shopland, D. R., Eyre, H.-J., and Pechacek, T.,** Smoking-attributable cancer mortality in 1991: is lung cancer now the leading cause of death among smokers in the United States?, *J. Natl. Cancer Inst.,* 83, 1142, 1991.

21. **Hoffmann, D., Djordjevic, M. V., and Brunnemann, K. D.,** Changes in cigarette design and composition over time and how they influence the yields of smoke constituents, *J. Smoking Relat. Disord.,* 6, 9, 1995.

22. **Bradford, J. A., Harlan, W. R., and Hanmer, H. R.,** Nature of cigarette smoke. Technique of experimental smoking, *Ind. Eng. Chem.,* 28, 836, 1936.

23. **Pillsbury, H. C., Bright, C. C., O'Connor, K. J., and Irish, F. W.,** Tar and nicotine in cigarette smoke, *J. Assoc. Off. Anal. Chem.,* 52, 458, 1969.

24. **U.S. Surgeon General,** The Health Consequences of Smoking. Nicotine Addiction, NIH Publ. No. 86-7874, 1986.

25. **Russell, M. A. H.,** The case for medium-nicotine, low-tar, low-carbon monoxide cigarettes, *Banbury Rep.,* 3, 297, 1980.

26. **Herning, R. I., Jones, R. T., Bachman, J., and Mines, A. H.,** Puff volume increases when low-nicotine cigarettes are smoked, *Br. Med. J. Clin. Res.,* 283, 187, 1981.

27. **Kozlowski, L. T., Rickert, W. S., Pope, M. A., Robinson, J. C., and Frecker, R. C.,** Estimating the yield to smokers of tar, nicotine, and carbon monoxide from the "lowest yield" ventilated filter-cigarettes, *Br. J. Addict.*, 77, 159, 1982.

28. **Fagerström, K. O.,** Effects of a nicotine enriched cigarette on nicotine titration, daily cigarette consumption and levels of carbon monoxide, cotinine and nicotine, *Psychopharmacology*, 77, 164, 1982.

29. **Haley, N. J., Sepkovic, D. W., Hoffmann, D., and Wynder, E. L.,** Cigarette smoking as a risk factor for cardiovascular disease. VI. Compensation with nicotine availability as a single variable, *Clin. Pharmacol. Ther.*, 38, 164, 1985.

30. **Puustinen, P., Olkkonen, H., Kolonen, S., and Tuomisto, J.,** Microcomputer-aided measurements of puff parameters during smoking of low- and medium-tar cigarettes, *Scand. J. Clin. Lab. Invest.*, 47, 655, 1987.

31. **Fischer, S., Spiegelhalder, B., and Preussmann, R.,** Influence of smoking parameters on the delivery of tobacco-specific nitrosamines in cigarette smoke: a contribution to relative risk evaluation, *Carcinogenesis*, 10, 1059, 1989.

32. **Djordjevic, M. V., Sigountos, C. W., Brunnemann, K. D., and Hoffmann, D.,** Tobacco-specific nitrosamine delivery in the mainstream smoke of high- and low-yield cigarettes smoked with varying puff volumes, Abstr. CORESTA Symp., Kallithea, Greece, 1990, 54.

33. **Lubin, J. H., Blot, W. J., Berrino, F., Flamant, R., Gillis, C. R., Kunze, M., Schmähl, D., and Visco, G.,** Patterns of lung cancer risk according to type of cigarette smoked, *Int. J. Cancer*, 33, 569, 1984.

34. **Rivenson, A., Hecht, S. S., and Hoffmann, D.,** Carcinogenicity of tobacco-specific *N*-nitrosoamines (TSNA): the role of the vascular network in the selection of target organs. *Crit. Rev. Toxicol.*, 21, 255, 1991.

35. **Hoffmann, D., Brunnemann, K. D., Prokopczyk, B., and Djordjevic, M. V.,** Tobacco-specific *N*-nitrosamines and areca-derived *N*-nitrosamines: chemistry, biochemistry, carcinogenicity, and relevance to humans, *J. Toxicol. Environ. Health*, 41, 1, 1994.

36. **LaVoie, E. J., Prokopczyk, B., Rigotty, J., Czech, A., Rivenson, A., and Adams, J. D.,** Tumorigenic activity of the tobacco-specific nitrosamines 4-(methylnitrosamino)-1-(3-pyridyl)-1-butanone (NNK), 4-(methylnitrosamino)-1-(3-pyridyl)-1-butanol (NNAL) and *N'*-nitrosonornicotine (NNN) on topical application to Sencar mice, *Cancer Lett.*, 37, 277, 1987.

37. **Hecht, S. S., Morse, M. A., Amin, S., Stoner, G. D., Jordan, K. G., Choi, C.-I., and Chung, F.-L.,** Rapid single-dose model for lung tumor induction in A/J mice by 4-(methylnitrosamino)-1-(3-pyridyl)-1-butanone and the effect of diet, *Carcinogenesis*, 10, 1901, 1989.

38. **Hoffmann, D., Djordjevic, M. V., Rivenson, A., Zang, E., Desai, D., and Amin, S.,** A study of tobacco carcinogenesis. LI. Relative potencies of tobacco-specific N-nitrosamines as inducers of lung tumors in A/J mice, *Cancer Lett.*, 71, 25, 1993.

39. **Hecht, S. S., Isaacs, S., and Trushin, N.,** Lung tumor induction in A/J mice by the tobacco smoke carcinogens 4-(methylnitrosamino)-1-(3-pyridyl)-1-butanone and benzo(a)pyrene: a potentially useful model for evaluation of chemopreventive agents, *Carcinogenesis*, 15, 2721, 1994.

40. **Anderson, L. M., Hecht, S. S., Kovatch, R. M., Amin, S., Hoffmann, D., and Rice, J. M.,** Tumorigenicity of the tobacco-specific carcinogen 4-(methylnitrosamino)-1-(3-pyridyl)-1-butanone in infant mice, *Cancer Lett.*, 58, 177, 1991.

41. **Prokopczyk, G., Rivenson, A., and Hoffmann, D.** A study of betel quid carcinogenesis. IX. Comparative carcinogenicity of 3-methylnitrosaminopropionitrile (MNPN) and 4-(methylnitrosamino)-1-(3-pyridyl)-1-butanone (NNK) upon local applications to mouse

skin and rat oral mucosa, *Cancer Lett.*, 60, 151, 1991.

42. **Lijinsky, W., Saavedra, J. E., and Kovatch, R. M.,** Carcinogenesis in rats by substituted dialkylnitrosamines given by gavage, *In Vivo*, 5, 85, 1991.

43. **Rivenson, A., Hoffmann, D., Prokopczyk, B., Amin, S., and Hecht, S. S.,** A study of tobacco carcinogenesis. XLII. Induction of lung and pancreas tumors in F344 rats by tobacco-specific and *areca*-derived *N*-nitrosamines, *Cancer Res.*, 48, 6912, 1988.

44. **Hecht, S. S., Chen, C.-H. B., Ohmori, T., and Hoffmann, D.,** Comparative carcinogenicity in F344 rats of the tobacco-specific nitrosamines, *N'*-nitrosonornicotine and 4-(N-methyl-N-nitrosamino)-1-(3-pyridyl)-1-butanone, *Cancer Res.*, 40, 298, 1980.

45. **Hoffmann, D., Rivenson, A., Amin, S., and Hecht, S. S.,** Dose-response study on the carcinogenicity of tobacco-specific *N*-nitrosamines in F344 rats, *J. Cancer Res. Clin. Oncol.*, 108, 81, 1984.

46. **Belinsky, S. A., Foley, J. F., White, C. M., Anderson, M. W., and Maronpot, R.,** Dose-response relationship between O^6-methylguanine formation on Clara cells and induction of pulmonary neoplasia in the rat by 4-(methylnitrosamino)-1-(3-pyridyl)-1-butanone, *Cancer Res.*, 50, 3772, 1990.

47. **Lijinsky, W., Thomas, B. J., and Kovatch, R. M.,** Local and systemic carcinogenic effects of alkylating carcinogens in rats treated with intravesicular administration, *Jpn. J. Cancer Res.*, 82, 980, 1991.

48. **Hoffmann, D., Castonguay, A., Rivenson, A., and Hecht, S. S.,** Comparative carcinogenicity and metabolism of 4-(methylnitrosamino)-1-(3-pyridyl)-1-butanone and *N'*-nitrosonornicotine in Syrian golden hamsters, *Cancer Res.*, 41, 2386, 1981.

49. **Hecht, S. S., Adams, J. D., Numoto, S., and Hoffmann, D.,** Induction of respiratory tract tumors in Syrian golden hamsters by a single dose of 4-(methylnitrosamino)-1-(3-pyridyl)-1-butanone (NNK) and the effect of smoke inhalation, *Carcinogenesis*, 4, 1287, 1983.

50. **Schuller, H. M., Witschi, H.-P., Nylen, E., Joshi, P. A., Correa, E., and Becker, K. L.,** Pathobiology of lung tumors induced in hamsters by 4-(methylnitrosamino)-1-(3-pyridyl)-1-butanone and the modulating effect of hyperoxia, *Cancer Res.*, 50, 1960, 1990.

51. **Oreffo, V. I. C., Lin, H.-W., Padmanabhan, R., and Witschi, H.,** K-ras and p53 point mutations in 4-(methylnitrosamino)-1-(3-pyridyl)-1-butanone-induced hamster lung tumors, *Carcinogenesis*, 14, 451, 1993.

52. **Hecht, S. S., Jordan, K. G., Choi, C.-I., and Trushin, N.,** Effects of deuterium substitution on the tumorigenicity of 4-(methylnitrosamino)-1-(3-pyridyl)-1-butanone and 4-(methylnitrosamino)-1-(3-pyridyl)-1-butanol in A/J mice, *Carcinogenesis*, 11, 1017, 1990.

53. **Boyland, E., Roe, J. C., and Gorrod, J. W.,** Induction of pulmonary tumors in mice by nitrosonornicotine, a possible constituent of tobacco smoke, *Nature*, 202, 1126, 1984.

54. **Hoffmann, D., Raineri, R., Hecht, S. S., Maronpot, R., and Wynder, E. L.,** A study of tobacco carcinogenesis. XIV. Effects of *N'*-nitrosonornicotine and *N'*-nitrosoanabasine in rats, *J. Natl. Cancer Inst.*, 55, 977, 1975.

55. **Hecht, S. S., Young, R., and Maeura, Y.,** Comparative carcinogenicity in F344 rats and Syrian golden hamsters of *N'*-nitrosonornicotine and *N'*-nitrosonornicotine-1-*N*-oxide, *Cancer Lett.*, 20, 333, 1983.

56. **Singer, G. M. and Taylor, H. W.,** Carcinogenicity of *N'*-nitrosonornicotine in Sprague-Dawley rats, *J. Natl. Cancer Inst.*, 57, 1275, 1976.

57. **Castonguay, A., Rivenson, A., Trushin, N., Reinhardt, J., Spathopoulos, S., Weiss, C., Reiss, B., and Hecht, S. S.,** Effects of

chronic ethanol consumption on the metabolism and carcinogenicity of N'-nitrosonornicotine in F344 rats, *Cancer Res.*, 44, 2285, 1984.

58. **Griciute, L., Castegnaro, M., Bereziat, J. C., and Cabral, J. R.,** Influences of ethyl alcohol on the carcinogenic activity of N-nitrosonornicotine, *Cancer Lett.*, 31, 267, 1986.

59. **Hilfrich, J., Hecht, S. S., and Hoffmann, D.,** A study of tobacco carcinogenesis. XV. Effects of N'-nitrosonornicotine and N'-nitrosoanabasine in Syrian golden hamsters, *Cancer Lett.*, 2, 169, 1977.

60. **McCoy, G. D., Hecht, S. S., Katayama, S., and Wynder, E. L.,** Differential effect of chronic ethanol consumption on the carcinogenicity of N-nitrosopyrrolidine and N'-nitrosonornicotine in male Syrian golden hamsters, *Cancer Res.*, 41, 2849, 1981.

61. **Koppang, N., Rivenson, A., Reith, A., Dahle, H. K., Evensen, O., and Hoffmann, D.,** A study of tobacco carcinogenesis. XLVIII. Carcinogenicity of N'-nitrosonornicotine in mink (Mustela vison), *Carcinogenesis*, 13, 1957, 1992.

62. **Boyland, E., Roe, F. J. C., Gorrod, J. W., and Mitchley, B. C. V.,** The carcinogenicity of nitrosoanabasine, a possible constituent of tobacco smoke, *Br. J. Cancer*, 18, 265, 1964.

63. **Brunnemann, K. D., Rivenson, A., Czech, A., LaVoie, E. J., and Hoffmann, D.,** Isolation, identification, and bioassay of the tobacco-specific N-nitrosamine 4-(methylnitrosamino)-1-(3-pyridyl)-1-butanol, *Proc. Am. Assoc. Cancer Res.*, 29, 84, 1988.

64. **Rivenson, A., Djordjevic, M. V., Amin, S., and Hoffmann, D.,** A study of tobacco carcinogenesis. XLIV. Bioassay in A/J mice of some N-nitrosamines, *Cancer Lett.*, 47, 111, 1989.

65. **Hecht, S. S. and Hoffmann, D.,** 4-(Methylnitrosamino)-1-(3-pyridyl)-1-butanone, a nicotine-derived tobacco-specific nitrosamine,

and cancer of the lung and pancreas in humans, in *Origin of Human Cancer. A. Comprehensive Review*, Brugge, J., Curran, T., Harlow, E., and McCormick, F., Eds., Cold Spring Harbor Laboratories, Cold Spring Harbor, NY, 1991, 745.

66. **Hecht, S. S. and Hoffmann, D.,** The relevance of tobacco-specific nitrosamines in human cancer, *Cancer Surv.*, 8, 273, 1989.

67. **Hecht, S. S., Trushin, N., Castonguay, A., and Rivenson, A.,** A comparative tumorigenicity of DNA methylation in F344 rats by 4-(methylnitrosamino)-1-(3-pyridyl)-1-butanone and N-nitrosomethylamine, *Cancer Res.*, 46, 498, 1986.

68. **Peterson, L. A. and Hecht, S. S.,** O^6-Methylguanine is a critical determinant of 4-(methylnitrosamino)-1-(3-pyridyl)-1-butanone tumorigenesis in A/J mouse lung, *Cancer Res.*, 51, 5557, 1991.

69. **Belinsky, S. A., Devereaux, T. R., Maronpot, R. R., Stoner, G. D., and Anderson, M. W.,** Relationship between the formation of promutagenic adducts and the activation of the K-ras protooncogene in lung tumors in A/J mice treated with nitrosamines, *Cancer Res.*, 49, 5305, 1989.

70. **Mustonen, R., Schoket, B., and Hemminki, K.,** Smoking-related DNA adducts: ^{32}P-postlabeling analysis of 7-methylguanine in human bronchial and lymphocyte DNA, *Carcinogenesis*, 14, 151, 1993.

71. **Foiles, P. G., Akerkar, S. A., Carmella, S. G., Kagan, M., Stoner, G. D., Resau, J. H., and Hecht, S. S.,** Mass spectrometric analysis of tobacco-specific nitrosamine-DNA adducts in smokers and nonsmokers, *Chem. Res. Toxicol.*, 4, 364, 1991.

72. **Rodenhuis, S. and Slebos, R. J. C.,** Clinical significance of ras oncogene activation in human lung cancer, *Cancer Res. Suppl.*, 52, 2665s, 1992.

73. **Kobayashi, T., Tsuda, H., Nognchi, M., Hirohashi, S., Shimosato, Y., Goya, T., and Hayata, Y.,** Association of point mutation in

c-Ki-ras oncogene in lung adenocarcinoma with particular reference to cytologic subtypes, *Cancer*, 66, 289, 1990.

74. **Belinsky, S. A., Devereaux, T. R., White, C. M., Foley, J. F., Maronpot, R. R., and Anderson, M. W.,** Role of Clara cells and type II cells in the development of pulmonary tumors in rats and mice following exposure to a tobacco-specific nitrosamine, *Exp. Lung Res.*, 17, 263, 1991.

75. **Ronai, Z. A., Gradia, S., Peterson, L. A., and Hecht, S. S.,** G to A transitions and G to T transversions in codon 12 of the Ki-ras oncogene isolated from mouse lung tumors induced by 4-(methylnitrosamino)-1-(3-pyridyl)-1-butanone (NNK) and related DNA methylating and pyridyloxobutylating agents, *Carcinogenesis*, 14, 2419, 1993.

76. **Hoffmann, D., Rivenson, A., Murphy, S. E., Chung, F.-L., Amin, S., and Hecht, S. S.,** Cigarette smoking and adenocarcinoma of the lung: the relevance of nicotine-derived *N*-nitrosamines, *J. Smoking-Relat. Disord.*, 4, 165, 1993.

COMPARATIVE CARCINOGENICITY, METABOLISM, MUTAGENICITY, AND DNA BINDING OF 7H-DIBENZO[c,g]CARBAZOLE AND DIBENZ[a,j]ACRIDINE

Critical Reviews in Toxicology, 26(2):213–249 (1996)

Comparative Carcinogenicity, Metabolism, Mutagenicity, and DNA Binding of 7H-Dibenzo[*c,g*]carbazole and Dibenz[*a,j*]acridine

David Warshawsky,* Glenn Talaska, Weiling Xue, and Joanne Schneider

Department of Environmental Health, University of Cincinnati, P.O. Box 670056, Cincinnati, OH 45267-0056

* To whom correspondence should be addressed.

ABSTRACT: Complex mixtures that are produced from the combustion of organic materials have been associated with increased cancer mortality. These mixtures contain homocyclic and heterocyclic polycyclic aromatic hydrocarbons (PAHs), many of which are known carcinogens. In particular, *N*-heterocyclic aromatic compounds (NHA) are present in these mixtures. Studies to determine the metabolic activation of these compounds have been undertaken. The purpose of this review is to compare and contrast the metabolic activation and biological effects of two NHA, 7H-dibenzo[*c,g*]carbazole (DBC) and dibenz[*a,j*]acridine (DBA), in order to better assess the contribution of NHA to the carcinogenic potency of complex mixtures and to develop biomarkers of the carcinogenic process. DBC has both local and systemic effects in the mouse; it is a potent skin and liver carcinogen following topical application and a lung carcinogen following i.p. application. On the other hand, DBA is a moderate mouse skin carcinogen following topical application and a lung carcinogen following subcutaneous injection. The biological differences for DBC and DBA are reflected in target organ-specific proximate and mutagenic metabolites and DNA adduct patterns.

KEY WORDS: 7H-dibenzo[*c,g*]carbazole; dibenz[*a,j*]acridine; *N*-heterocyclic aromatic compounds; DNA binding, metabolism, carcinogenicity; mutagenicity; organotropism.

I. INTRODUCTION

Exposure to complex mixtures resulting from combustion processes such as soot, coal tar and pitch, mineral oils, and coal gasification residues has been associated with increased cancer mortality.[1–7] These mixtures contain polynuclear aromatic compounds that are released into the environment from sources ranging from smoke stack and coke oven effluents to tobacco smoke; the carcinogenicity of these mixtures is well recognized.[1–7] Studies of the PAH fractions have been the primary focus of efforts to define the carcinogenicity of mixtures.[2,3,4,8–10] Benzo[*a*]pyrene (BaP) has been the best-characterized PAH as a potential indicator of biological activity of the PAH fraction.[2] NHAs have been identified in neutral and basic fractions of complex mixtures from motor vehicle exhaust,[11] effluents from coal and oil processing,[12] coke oven emissions,[13] coal tar-based therapeutic agents,[14] tobacco smoke condensates,[15] carbon black emissions,[16] synthetic fuels,[17] sea water,[18] industrial and urban atmospheres,[19,20] and coal gasification residues.[21] Based on the contribution of NHA to complex mixtures, we have attempted to study the metabolic activation of NHA. In particular, we selected DBC and DBA (Figure 1) as model compounds for our studies based on animal testing of members of that class of compounds, much of which was done between 1930 and 1950. Both DBC and DBA were found to be carcinogenic in more than one tissue. Additionally, both compounds were symmetric around their C_2 axis, with the only difference being that the middle ring for DBC had a pyrrole ring whereas DBA had a pyridine ring. Therefore, it was hoped that the information obtained could be used to develop a structure-activity relationship for NHA. This review addresses what is known about DBC and DBA, and compares and contrasts the results obtained for their carcinogenicity, metabolism, mutagenicity, and DNA binding.

II. CARCINOGENICITY

NHAs have been studied for the past 60 years.[1] DBC has been shown to be a potent carcinogen to mouse skin and mouse liver by topical application and subcutaneous injection as well as being a pulmonary and forestomach carcinogen in mouse following subcutaneous injection and oral administration, respectively.[22–30] DBC was also shown to be carcinogenic in mouse lung following intravenous injection[31] and in mouse liver following intraperitoneal administration.[32] DBC was carcinogenic in the urinary bladder of the dog following intravesical injection[33] and in the rat following subcutaneous injection.[23] DBC was carcinogenic in hamster lung with and with-

out carrier dust, ferric oxide,[34–36] following intratracheal administration. Using doses comparable to BaP plus ferric oxide, DBC plus ferric oxide was more carcinogenic in the hamster lung.[37] In summary, DBC was carcinogenic in mouse, rat, hamster, and dog, with both local and systemic effects (Table 1).

On the other hand, DBA was found to be a moderate to weakly active carcinogen to mouse skin by topical application and subcutaneous injection.[38–42] DBA was also carcinogenic in mouse lung following subcutaneous injection.[31] However, DBA was not active in the hamster and rat lung following either intratracheal administration or injection into the lung, respectively.[43,44] Similarly, when DBA and ferric oxide were given together intratracheally to hamsters, no effect was seen[44] (Table 2).

In order to begin our work on the metabolic activation of DBC and DBA, we felt it was necessary to assess DBC and DBA in the mouse skin model in a complete carcinogenesis protocol as well as in an initiation-promotion protocol. This reasoning was based on our evaluation of earlier studies that displayed several shortcomings: the purity of the compound was not always reported, benzene was used as a solvent in some cases, toxic doses were used in several instances, and an inadequate number of controls were used in many cases. Second, it was important to compare the carcinogenicity of these two compounds to each other as well as to a third, well-known carcinogen, BaP, because up to that point no such study had been undertaken.

The sources and purity of DBC, DBA, and BaP were reported.[45] DBC was synthesized in the laboratory and purified by recrystallization to greater than 99% purity. Both DBA and BaP were purchased with 99% purity and were further purified to 99.5% purity by column chromatography in conjunction with recrystallization. The

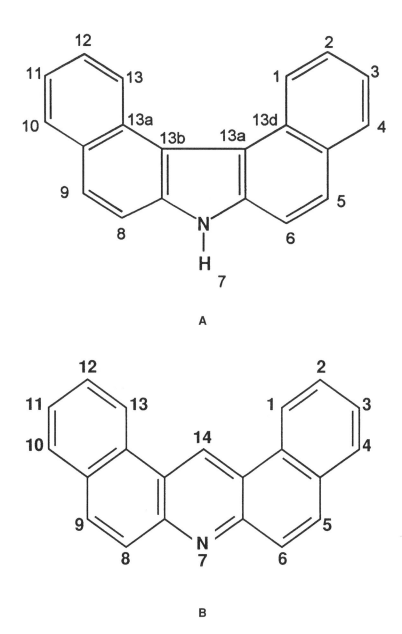

FIGURE 1. Structure of (A) 7H-dibenzo[*c,g*]carbazole (DBC) and (B) dibenz[*a,j*]acridine (DBA).

purity of all three compounds was monitored by high-performance liquid chromatography (HPLC), UV, and mass spectrometry.

This laboratory has a long history of using mouse skin carcinogenicity studies to examine the mechanism of action of a variety of compounds and materials, such as PAHs, coal tar, asphalt, and various petroleum and shale oil products.[2-4] The C3H mouse was the model of choice for the mixtures and compounds mentioned above. Thus, although the C3H mouse appeared to be less sensitive in complete carcinogenicity and in initiation-promotion studies, it was the animal of choice in our first study due the historical database.[46] Based on the fact that solutions of 0.1 to 0.5% for DBC and DBA were toxic in prior studies, 50 male C3H mice per group were treated twice

TABLE 1
Tumor Studies for DBC

Type	Sex	No.	Total dose (mg)	Mode of administration	Time range	Observation	Ref.
Simpson strain	—	26[a]	4.2–4.8	0.3% reduced to 0.1% in benzene skin painting, ×2w	100–321 d	4 carcinoma skin[b] 4 papilloma skin	23
Simpson strain	—	25[c]	2.4–6.2	0.1% skin painting in benzene, ×2w	150–321 d	4 carcinoma skin[b] 5 hepatomas[d]	23
CBA	M	5	—	0.5% skin painting in benzene, ×2w	several months	4 s.c. carcinomas	24
CBA	M	18	1.2	6 s.c. injection of 0.2 ml of 0.1% solution in sesame oil weekly	204 d	14 s.c. sarcomas 5 hepatomas 2 pulmonary tumors	24
CBA	M	24	1.2	6 s.c. injection of 0.2 ml of 0.1% solution in sesame oil weekly	145 d	24 s.c. sarcomas 3 hepatomas	24
A	M	18	1.2	6 s.c. injection of 0.2 ml of 0.1% solution in sesame oil weekly	138 d	17 s.c. sarcomas	24
Stock mouse	—	28	0.25	1 i.p. injection of 12.5 mg/kg/bw in olive oil	176 d	1 sarcoma at site[e] of injection	32
Stock mouse	—	83	0.25	1 i.p. injection of 12.5 mg/kg/bw in olive oil	35–200 d	33 bile duct proliferation or cholangiomas	32
A	F	20	0.2	1 s.c. injection of 0.2 mg in sesame oil	280 d	17 sarcomas 8 lung tumors	31
A	M and F	10	0.25	0.25 µg in aqueous suspension given i.v.	56 d	7 lung tumors[f]	
A	M and F	10	0.25	0.25 µg in aqueous suspension given i.v.	98 d	9 lung tumors[f]	
A	M and F	12	0.25	0.25 µg in aqueous suspension given i.v.	140 d	12 lung tumors[f]	
A	F	170	0.2	0.2 mg in lard, sesame oil, or olive oil s.c. injection	10–42 weeks	116 pulmonary tumors 62 s.c. sarcomas	30

Strain	Sex	No.	Dose	Treatment	Duration	Tumours	Ref.
A	M	83	0.2	0.2 mg in lard, sesame oil, or olive oil s.c. injection	10–42 weeks	47 s.c. sarcomas	
CH$_3$	F	11	0.2	0.2 mg in lard, sesame oil, or olive oil s.c. injection	10–42 weeks	5 s.c. sarcomas	
CH$_3$	M	49	0.2	0.2 mg in lard, sesame oil, or olive oil s.c. injection	10–42 weeks	22 s.c. sarcomas	
C	F	23	0.2	0.2 mg in lard, sesame oil, or olive oil s.c. injection	10–42 weeks	11 s.c. sarcomas	
C	M	44	0.2	0.2 mg in lard, sesame oil, or olive oil s.c. injection	10–42 weeks	35 s.c. sarcomas	
A	M and F	24	14–23	0.25–4.0 mg as a 0.125–1% solution in arachis oil by stomach tube; ×2w	17–59 weeks	17 forestomach pap, 3 forestomach carc, 4 benign hepatoma, 18 malignant hepatomas[e]	22
CBA	M and F	31	7–23	0.25–4.0 mg as a 0.125–1% solution in arachis oil by stomach tube; ×2w	17–59 weeks	24 pulmonary adeno, 18 forestomach pap, 4 forestomach carc, 15 benign hepatomas, 1 malignant hepatoma[g]	
Stock mouse	M and F	24	ND	0.1–0.2% solution in acetone (1 or 2 weeks); topical application	550 d	5 papillomas, 12 carcinomas	25
Stock mouse	M and F	20	0.2–0.4	0.2–0.4 mg in arachis oil; single injection	280 d	12 sarcomas, 1 hepatoma[h]	
CBA	M and F	12	ND	0.2% solution in acetone; topical application, x3w	110 d	papillomas, squamous carcinomas, and 1 hepatoma[i]	26
CBA	M and F	10	0.8	0.3 mg in 0.25 ml tricaprylin plus 0.5 mg in 0.25 ml arachis oil; single injections	110 d	8 sarcomas[i], 2 hepatomas	

TABLE 1 (continued)
Tumor Studies for DBC

Type	Sex	No.	Total dose (mg)	Mode of administration	Time range	Observation	Ref.
Stock mouse	M and F	15	3	3 s.c. injections of 1 mg in arachis oil over 1–month period	240–382 d	7 developed sarcomas[j]	29
C₃H	M	50	0.9	12.5 μg topically in acetone ×2w	364	48 skin tumors 47 carcinomas 1 papilloma	46
Hsd:ICR-(Br)	F	50	1.47	13.3 μg topically in acetone ×2w	560	37 liver tumors, mostly hepatocellular adenomas and carcinomas 42 skin tumors, majority squamous cell carcinomas	47
Hsd:ICR-(Br)	F	30	0.053	53.2 μg topically once, followed 2 weeks later by TPA, 2 μg x ×2w for 24 weeks	182	26 mice with papillomas	48
Mouse	—	14	1–2	Implantation of 10–20 mg paraffin wax pellets containing 1–2 mg to bladder	98	3 papillomas or adenomas 2 carcinomas 2 metaplasia[k]	27
A/J mouse	M	80	40, 20, 10, 5 mg/kg bw; 20 per dose	i.p. injection in 0.2 ml tricaprylin	240	Lung tumor response dose related, with average 4.7 ± 1.2 tumors per mouse at 5 mg/kg and 48.1 and 5.5 tumors per mouse at 40 mg/kg (control: 0.6 ± 0.6 lung tumors)	49
Rat	—	10	5.6	0.05% colloidal suspension, 2ml x ×2w	196	8 sarcomas	23
Syrian golden hamster	M	35	45	15 weekly instillations in lung of 3 mg suspended with equal amounts of hematite in saline	105	86% had respiratory tract tumors; of the tumor-bearing animals, 50% had squamous cell carcinomas of bronchial and tracheal epithelium	34

Species	Sex			Treatment		Results	
Syrian golden hamster	M	45	15	30 weekly instillations in lung of 0.5 mg suspended with equal amounts of hematite in saline	210	89% had respiratory tract tumors; 64% of animals bore a total of 51 squamous cell carcinomas of trachea, bronchi, and larynx	
Syrian golden hamster	M	46	9	18 weekly installations in lung at 0.5 mg per dose in 0.2 ml water	490	33 developed respiratory tract tumors	36
Syrian golden hamster	M	45	30	3-mg weekly instillations in lung for 10 weeks in 0.2 ml water	490	15 developed[i] respiratory tract tumors; in both groups, tumors were mainly papillomas, squamous cell carcinomas, and adenocarcinomas, mainly in trachea and bronchi	
Dog	F	4	90	5 ml of 0.25% solution in arachis oil administered to bladder for 12 months	1230	One developed approx. 40 papillomas and one urinary transitional-cell carcinoma[m]	33

a   Thirty-four died early.

b   Eighty percent of those who survived a month showed hypertrophic biliary changes estimates of 0.8 mg to produce biliary changes and 6 mg for hepatoma.

c   Five died early.

d   No hepatomas in 35 controls.

e   Twenty-eight of 65 survived 39 d.

f   Controls: 1/20, 3/20, and 4/19 lung tumors.

g   Controls not reported.

h   Twelve survived 100 d.

i   Eight survived.

j   Seven survived.

k   Six did not survive.

l   Toxicity.

m   One survived to develop tumors.

TABLE 2
Tumor Studies for DBA

Type	Sex	No.	Total dose (mg)	Route of administration	Time range (d)	Observation	Ref.
Mouse	ND	10	ND	5 mg given weekly in olive oil orally or by stomach tube in butter	572	No tumors	38
Mouse	ND	40	ND	0.3% solution in benzene; topical application, ×2w	597	11 squamous cell carcinomas 2 papillomas	
Mouse	ND	10	ND	Repeated s.c. injections of 5 mg in sesame oil	583	2 sarcomas	
Mouse	ND	40	ND	0.3% solution in benzene; topical application, ×2w	551–597	2 papillomas[a] 11 squamous cell carcinomas	39
XVII mouse	ND	20	ND	0.3% solution in acetone; topical application, one drop twice weekly	402	No tumors	40
XVII mouse	ND	10	3	0.5–1 mg in arachis oil; 3 s.c. injections at 1-month intervals	590	No tumors	
Mouse	ND	20	ND	0.1% solution in acetone; topical application, ×3w	420	15 tumors	42
Mouse	ND	20	ND	0.5% solution in acetone; topical application, ×3w	420	16 tumors; 60% of both group carcinomas	
A	ND	13	1.0	Single s.c. injection, 1 mg in 0.3 ml sesame oil	280	No sarcomas 13 lung tumors[b]	31
Mouse	ND	20	0.022	0.3 ml of 0.3% of solution in sesame oil every 2 weeks; s.c. injection	266–310	No tumors	41

C₃H	M	50	2	12.5 µg in 50 µl acetone; topical application, ×2w	693	25 tumors 3 papillomas 22 carcinomas	46
Hsd:ICR-(Br)	F	50	1.74	13.95 µg in 50 µl acetone; topical application, ×2w	693	27 skin tumors 15 squamous cell carcinomas 7 papillomas 3 basal cell carcinomas	47
Hsd:ICR-(Br)	F	30	0.056	55.8 µg in 50 µl acetone once, followed 2 weeks later by TPA, ×2w, for 24 weeks	182	17 mice with papillomas	48

a   Twenty-one survived 1 year; 34 survived 6 months.

b   Four single lung tumors developed in 18 controls.

a week with 12.5 μg (0.025% solution) of BaP (49.6 nmol), DBC (46.8 nmol), or DBA (44.8 nmol) delivered in 50 μl of acetone to the interscapular region of the back. An acetone group of 50 mice received 50 μl of distilled acetone twice weekly. A no-treatment group of 50 animals was also included. Applications were continued for 99 weeks or until the animal became moribund. Both DBC and BaP produced 48 skin tumors in 50 mice, of which 47 in each group were squamous cell carcinomas and one papilloma, while DBA produced 25 tumors, of which 22 were squamous cell carcinomas and 3 papillomas. The latency periods for DBC, BaP, and DBA were 36.6, 32.4, and 80 weeks, respectively. Based on the latency and tumor incidence, DBC was found to be as potent a skin carcinogen as BaP and more so than DBA. No liver tumors were found for DBC, probably due to the rapid appearance of malignant skin tumors. No tumors were seen in the acetone or no-treatment groups.[46]

The next two studies involved using a strain more sensitive to skin carcinogenesis, the Hsd:ICR(BR) mouse, that was equivalent to the CD-1 mouse. The rationale used was that this strain showed a good correlation between the tumor-initiating activity of PAHs and NHA and their ability to covalently bind to DNA, and this strain had been used in several metabolism and DNA binding studies that had been reported in the literature.[47] In a complete carcinogenicity study, 50 nmol of DBC, DBA, BaP, or DBC plus BaP (25 nmol + 25 nmol) were applied to the shaved backs of 50 female Hsd:ICR(BR) mice per group twice a week in 50 μl of acetone for 99 weeks or until the appearance of a tumor. Fifty mice each were used in two control groups: acetone and no-treatment groups. The histopathology data indicated primary skin lesions in 42, 27, 48, and 47 of 50 mice each for DBC, DBA, BaP, and DBC plus DBA, respectively, the

majority of them being squamous cell carcinomas. In addition, primary liver lesions were present in 37 mice in the DBC group; 17 of the lesions were hepatocellular adenomas and 22 were hepatocellular carcinomas with only slight necrosis in only five animals, of which only one had a liver lesion. The no-treatment group had two animals with skin lesions, but no squamous cell carcinomas, and one animal with a liver lesion with one hepatocellular adenoma. The acetone-treatment group had three animals with skin lesions, with one squamous cell carcinoma, and two animals with liver lesions, with a total of two hepatocellular adenomas. Coincident with the tumor data, the morphological and morphometric data indicated a significant increase ($p < 0.05$) in mononuclear cells in the dermis for the BaP and DBC plus BaP groups relative to the control (non-treated plus acetone-treated) group. Significant increases ($p < 0.05$) were observed in the nuclear area, nucleoli per nucleus, and cellular area of hepatocytes in the DBC-treatment group relative to the control group. These data indicated that DBC was a two-target organ carcinogen, a potent liver as well as a skin carcinogen following topical application with noted changes in the liver, whereas BaP was only a potent skin carcinogen and DBA a moderate skin carcinogen. It should also be noted that BaP produced skin tumors with a shorter latency period than DBC or DBA in this mouse strain. With this strain, skin tumors appeared more slowly for DBC than with the C3H strain, thus allowing for the appearance of liver tumors beginning around 45 to 50 weeks.

In a second study, the initiating ability for DBC and DBA was determined in the Hsd:ICR(Br) mouse strain using an initiation-promotion skin protocol.[48] 12-*O*-Tetradecanoylphorbol-13-acetate (TPA)- and BaP-treated animals were used as promoter and initiator only controls, respectively. No-treatment animals were also included. DBC, DBA, or BaP (200 nmol) dissolved in acetone was applied once to the shaved backs of 30 mice, followed 2 weeks later with 2 μg of TPA in 50 μl of acetone applied twice a week for up to 24 weeks. Papillomas developed in 26, 17, and 27 animals, respectively. DBC plus TPA produced a significant influx of dermal macrophages similar to that seen for BaP plus TPA. Initiation with DBC, DBA, or BaP modulated the effect of TPA on most other dermal parameters, particularly neutrophils. Mice treated with BaP, DBC, DBA, TPA, or no-treatment only did not produce tumors in the skin. These data indicated that DBC showed tumor-initiating ability and morphological changes similar to that of BaP.

Finally, we undertook a study to determine whether tissue specificity for DBC lung carcinogenicity in the strain A/J mouse was mirrored by the formation of DBC-DNA adducts in the lung tissue, and whether these adducts were consistent with mutation patterns in the K-*ras* gene.[49] Strain A/J mice were given a single i.p. injection of DBC at doses of 0, 5, 10, 20, or 40 mg/kg, and the lungs were monitored for DNA adducts on days 1, 3, 5, 7, 14, and 21. The remaining animals were sacrificed 8 months after DBC treatment. The lung tumor response to DBC was dose related, with an average of 4.7 ± 1.2 tumors per mouse at 5 mg/kg and 48.1 ± 5.5 tumors per mouse at 40 mg/kg. As many as seven adducts were seen in the lung and liver. DNA-binding levels in the lung were highest at 40 mg/kg, with maximum binding at 5 to 7 d. At lower dose levels, the maximum binding to DNA decreased and shifted to earlier time points. Although the binding levels in the liver were ten times the levels in the lung, no tumors were seen at 8 months, but similar shifts in time of maximum binding of DBC to DNA to earlier time points were

observed. The major adduct in the lung was different from that seen in the liver (see section V for more details). The majority of DBC-induced mutations in the K-*ras* gene in the lung were A → T (76%) transversions in the third base of the 61st codon (Table 3), a mutation that has not been seen before in chemically induced lung tumors in the strain A/J mouse. These data suggested that DBC was a potent lung carcinogen in the strain A/J mouse and that the major DBC-DNA lung adduct may be the major promutagen, consistent with specific K-*ras* mutations in the lung.

III. METABOLISM

A. Metabolism of DBA

The metabolism of DBA has been studied in some detail both *in vitro* and *in vivo*. We first investigated DBA in an isolated perfused rabbit lung preparation.[50] The rate of the metabolism of DBA was less than the rate of metabolism of DBC (see below) in the corn oil-pretreated animals. With BaP-pretreated animals, the rate of metabolism was markedly (fivefold) increased over corn oil controls. Combining HPLC separation with UV, fluorescence spectroscopy, and mass spectrometry, one of the major organic solvent-soluble metabolites was assigned as 3,4-dihydrodiol-DBA, and another one was identified as a hydroxyl derivative of DBA. Later, using authentic synthetic standards[51] with an HPLC-UV photodiode array or fluorescence techniques and mass spectrometry, the metabolism of DBA in liver and lung microsomal preparations from 3-MC-pretreated rats was examined.[45,52–54] *Trans*-3,4-dihydroxy-3,4-dihydro-DBA (3,4-dihydrodiol-DBA), *trans*-5,6-dihydroxy-5,6-dihydro-DBA (5,6-dihydrodiol-DBA), DBA-5,6-oxide, 3-hydroxy-DBA, 4-hydroxy-DBA, and DBA-*N*-oxide were

TABLE 3
Mutation Spectra of the *K-ras* Gene in DBC-Induced Lung Tumors Compared with Spontaneous Lung Adenomas in Strain A/J Mice[a]

K-*ras* mutations

| Treatment | No. of tumors | Codon 12 | | | | | Codon 61 | | | | Total |
		CGT→Gly[b]	TGT CyS	GTT Val	CGT Arg	GAT Asp	CAA→Gln	CAT His	CTA Leu	CGA Arg	
Spontaneous	10	—	0	2	1	3	—	1	0	2	9 (90%)
DBC (all tumors)	49	—	0	0	0	0	—	35	9	2	46 (94%)

a   Sequencing analyses from DNA of lung adenomas from all four dose groups.[49]

b   The amino acid that is encoded for by normal or mutated codon directly above.

identified metabolites. Among them, 3,4-dihydrodiol, the candidate proximate carcinogen according to the bay-region theory, appeared to be the most prominent metabolite (30 to 40%), and 5,6-oxide was found to be the second major metabolite. The further oxidized (secondary) metabolites, such as 5,6-8,9-dioxide, tetrols, diolepoxides, and phenolic dihydrodiols, were also present.[52] For comparison with an isomer of DBA, the metabolism of dibenz[c,h]acridine (DB[c,h]A) by rat liver microsomes produced 10 to 17% of the trans-3,4-dihydrodiol-DB[c,h]A, which was further metabolized to the bay-region DB[c,h]A-3,4-dihydrodiol 1,2-epoxide to an extent of 15 to 23%.[55] Although the synthesized DBA-3,4-dihydrodiol 1,2-epoxide was available,[51] the direct evidence of its presence as a metabolite of DBA by 3-MC-pretreated rat liver microsomes has not yet been confirmed.[52,56] It should be noted that the 3,4-dihydrodiol of DBA was the major metabolite produced from the incubation of DBA with human liver microsomes.[57] This metabolite was formed by human microsomes P4501A1, -1A2, -3A4, and -3A5, with the highest relative amount formed by P4503A4.[58]

Similar to the metabolism observed for BaP, pretreatment of both mice and rats with 3-MC resulted in significant increases in the liver microsomal metabolism of DBA to dihydrodiols and phenols relative to corn oil treatment.[45] Additional comparative studies were carried out on the metabolism of DBA using liver preparations induced by five different chemicals (3-MC, Aroclor 1254, DBA, DBC, and phenobarbital) in order to assess whether the metabolism of DBA involved both PAH and aromatic amine biotransformation. 3-MC was used as an effective inducer of PAH metabolism (20 mg/kg on two successive days in corn oil), phenobarital as an effective inducer of aromatic amine metabolism (75 mg/kg on four successive days in saline), Aroclor 1254 as an effective inducer of a multitude of compounds, including PAH and aromatic amine metabolism (500 mg/kg once in corn oil), and DBC and DBA as potential inducers of NHA metabolism (20 mg/kg on two sucessive days in corn oil) relative to the corn oil control (2 ml/kg on two sucessive days).[59,60] Male Sprague-Dawley rats and female Hsd:ICR (Br) mice were pretreated, and liver microsomal and S-9 preparations were made. The following points were observed:

1. Metabolism of DBA by rat and mouse liver microsomes resulted in markedly higher total metabolites than the corresponding rat and mouse S-9 preparations. Except for Aroclor 1254, pretreated mouse S-9 and rat and mouse S-9 preparations did not increase the metabolism of DBA compared with the corn oil control (Table 4).

2. 3-MC-, Aroclor 1254-, and DBA-pretreated rat microsomes and 3-MC- and Aroclor 1254-pretreated mouse microsomes showed increased activity in metabolizing DBA relative to the corn oil control, while DBC and phenobarbital were inactive as inducers in both cases and DBA was inactive in the case of mouse microsomes (Table 4).

3. Different metabolite profiles were observed in the metabolism by 3-MC-pretreated rat or mouse microsomes. The ratio of 3,4-dihydrodiol to the 5,6-dihydrodiol by rat microsomes was approximately 2:1, and 1,2-dihydrodiol was about 5.5% of the total radioactivity, whereas with 3MC mouse microsomes, these values were 10:1 and 1.5%, respectively.

4. In summary, these studies indicated that DBA was metabolized by a set of similar enzymes that metabolized other PAHs in both rat and mouse.[45,59,60]

TABLE 4
Quantitation of Total Metabolism of DBA by Rat or Mouse Microsomes or S-9 with Different Inducers

% metabolism[a,b]

Preparation	Corn oil	3-MC	Aroclor	DBA	DBC	PB
Rat mic.	39.4 + 5.7[c]	57.2 + 15.6[c]*	50.1 + 10.9*	45.0 + 2.8[d]*	41.3 + 2.8[e]	38.2 + 1.6[f]
Rat S-9	24.8 + 3.2	26.0 + 3.1	32.7 + 5.2	27.6 + 3.6	27.0 + 2.5	30.4 + 2.7
Mouse mic.	32.1 + 4.3	50.6 + 14.2*	57.2**	31.2 + 5.2*	23.8 + 2.2 *	29.7 + 5.2*
Mouse S-9	25.7 + 3.0*	29.8 + 0.8*	49.2 + 3.9[g]	25.2 + 4.6	—	—

a Mean percent of all metabolites as a function of total radioactivity ± SD, n = 3; *n = 4, **n = 1.

b All microsomal and S-9 incubations with ^{14}C-DBA or ^{14}C-DBC contained 0.24 μmol substrate/sample (0.41 μCi/μmol) and NADPH-regenerating system and total protein of 1.6 mg in a total value of 4 ml. The reaction mixture was incubated at 37°C for 1 h.[45]

c Rat microsomes significantly greater than rat S-9 and mouse S-9 at $p \leq 0.05$.

d Rat microsomes significantly greater than rat S-9, mouse S-9, and mouse microsomes at $p \leq 0.05$.

e Rat microsomes significantly greater than rat S-9 and mouse microsomes at $p \leq 0.05$.

f Rat microsomes significantly greater than mouse microsomes at $p \leq 0.05$.

g Aroclor mouse S-9 is greater than corn oil, 3-MC, or DBA S-9 at $p \leq 0.05$.

For quantitation of metabolites, radiolabeled DBA (^{3}H or ^{14}C) was usually used. A nonradiometric technique[53] using synchronous fluorescence spectroscopy (SFS), which gave a single peak for each metabolite, was developed in order to reduce the use of radiolabeled materials. Regression equations of the SFS peak area vs. concentrations of the synthetic standards were employed to calculate the quantities of the metabolites produced in the metabolism studies. These values were in agreement with those obtained from radioactivity measurements.

Applying organic synthesis techniques and the techniques of separation of diastereoisomers, chiral stationary-phase chromatography, circular dichroic (CD) spectroscopy, and 1H nuclear magnetic resonance (NMR), the absolute configurations of the major metabolites 3,4-dihydrodiol-DBA and DBA-5,6-oxide were studied and assigned.[61] The enantiomeric composition of *trans*-3,4-dihydrodiol-DBA formed as microsomal metabolites of corn oil rat liver preparations was determined to be 69% 3 (R), 4 (R)-diol-DBA. When 3-MC-pretreated rat liver microsomes were used, the percentage was found to be 70% for the 3 (R), 4 (R)-diol-DBA (essentially no change). DBA-5,6-oxide formed as microsomal metabolites by corn oil rat liver preparations was determined to be 81% 5 (R), 6 (S)-oxide-DBA. However, when 3-MC-pretreated rat liver microsomes were used, the percentage was found to be 5% for DBA-5(R),6(S)-oxide. The data indicated a reversed stereochemical preference for oxide formation by the 3-MC-induced rat liver microsomes.

In order to assess DBA metabolism *in vivo*, the following studies were undertaken to corroborate the *in vitro* data. Phase II metabolites — water-soluble conjugates (glutathiones, sulfates, and glucuronides) — were also found to be distributed in blood

and lung.[50,62] Using ^{3}H-DBA, the metabolism of DBA *in vivo* in rats showed rapid excretion into the bile in 6 h following i.p. administration of 0.5 mg/kg and i.v. doses of 0.5 mg/kg.[63] After β- glucuronidase and arylsulfatase hydrolysis, approximately 25% of the biliary radioactivity was soluble in ethyl acetate. The organic solvent-soluble fraction contained \more secondary polar metabolites and approximately 1 to 2% 3,4-dihydrodiol-DBA by HPLC analysis. Without enzymatic hydrolysis, only 3% of the total radioactivity was ethyl acetate soluble. After topical application of ^{3}H-DBA to mice,[64] the levels of radioactivity were highest in the kidney at 6 h and the liver at 12 h. The total radioactivity in skin decreased from 87 to 46% over 96 h. In the liver after 48 h, the proportion of parent DBA was 25 to 30%, and two metabolites tentatively identified as 1,2-diol-DBA and 3,4-diol-DBA comprised 2 to 6% of the total radioactivity. Two less polar metabolites that were not identified comprised 2.5% of the total activity in the skin and 5 to 16% in the liver.

In conclusion, for the metabolism of DBA both *in vivo* and *in vitro*, in rat, mouse, and human, the dihydrodiols were the major products, and the 3,4-dihydrodiol was the most abundant.

B. Metabolism of DBC

DBC was unusual in its carcinogenic response following topical application in mouse in that it was potent both at the site of application and at a distant site,[47] namely, liver. The metabolism of DBC, unlike many of the PAHs such as BaP and DBA, by rodent liver cells, liver microsomes, and rabbit lung preparations showed that phenols were the predominant metabolites rather than dihydrodiols.[45,53,65–67] The ultimate carcinogenic metabolites of DBC are not clearly identified as yet.[68] Among the phenolic metabolites identified, 5-OH-DBC was the major one, comprising of 30 to 60% of the total metabolites formed by 3-MC-pre-treated rat liver microsomes, followed by 3-OH-DBC and other monohydroxy derivatives. However, although the parent DBC was sarcomagenic, both 5-OH-DBC and 3-OH-DBC were not sarcomagenic following subcutaneous injection, and only 3-OH-DBC showed slight hepatocarcinogenicity following i.p. injections.[68] It was expected that DBC would be metabolized through an *N*-hydroxyl intermediate,[66,68] as is the case for the hepatoactive aromatic amines.[69,70] This assumption was supported by the lack of carcinogenicity in the liver for *N*-methyl-DBC, whose nitrogen at the seven position is blocked with a methyl group.[71] Probably due to the extreme instability of the *N*-OH-DBC, the synthesis of this compound was not successful,[68,72] although most of the monohydroxylated derivatives of DBC were made available.[65,67,72] Acetylation stabilized the monohydroxylated derivatives of DBC and confirmed the existence of 1-OH-DBC, 2-OH-DBC, and 6,6′-*bis*-(5-OH-DBC) besides 5-OH-DBC and 3-OH-DBC in the metabolism products formed by 3-MC-treated rat liver microsomes; *N*-OH-DBC was not detected.[73]

3-MC-treated rat liver microsomes significantly increased DBC metabolism relative to corn oil control, whereas this was not the case with similarly pretreated mouse liver microsomes.[45] With Aroclor 1254 as the inducer, DBC was metabolized more readily by pretreated microsomes than by corn oil control.[74] The metabolic profiles formed by these preparations appeared to be dependent upon the enzyme inducers used as well as the substrate, proteins, and their concentrations. Studies of the metabolism of DBC, similar to that previously mentioned for DBA, by liver microsomal and S-9 preparations of male Sprague-Dawley rats and female Hsd:ICR (Br) mice pretreated with 3-MC, Aroclor, DBA, DBC,

phenobarbital, and corn oil control showed the following points:

1. 3-MC-, Aroclor 1254-, and DBA-pretreated rat microsomes and 3-MC-, Aroclor 1254-, and PB-treated rat S-9 preparations significantly increased DBC metabolism compared with corn oil controls. The remaining pretreatments of rat livers and all pretreatments of mice did not produce significant differences compared with corn oil controls (Table 5).

2. Metabolism by 3-MC-induced rat liver microsomes produced 5-OH-DBC as the major metabolite, while 3-OH-DBC seemed to be the major metabolite formed from the corresponding induced S-9 preparations (Table 6). These data suggested that induced rat microsomes had an effect on DBC metabolism, and more so than induced mouse microsomes, which may have an important role in the metabolic activation and carcinogenic endpoint of DBC in these two rodent models. This research awaits further investigation.

Very little work has been carried out *in vivo* for DBC. Several studies were undertaken to corroborate the *in vitro* data. In an *in vivo* study using ^{3}H-DBC applied topically at doses of 45.7, 106.7, and 145.7 nmol, there was a linear increase of radioactivity in the kidney, liver, lung, and spleen over time up to 48 h.[64] In the kidney the levels of radioactivity were highest at 6 and 12 h. After HPLC separation of the ethyl acetate extract of the skin and liver, the percents of total radioactivity for DBC and metabolites were determined. The proportion of DBC as parent compound decreased from 87 to 35% in the skin over 48 h and the proportion of parent DBC in the liver was 10%. Two metabolites tentatively identified as 3-OH-DBC and 5-OH-

TABLE 5
Quantitation of Total Metabolism of DBC by Rat or Mouse Microsomes or S-9 with Different Inducers

Preparation	% metabolism[a,b]				
	Corn oil	3-MC	Aroclor	DBA	DBC	PB
Rat mic.	30.6 + 3.7	59.1 + 1.8[c,f]	50.0 + 3.9[c,g]	53.4 + 5.3[c,h]	29.2 + 4.2	33.9 + 3.5
Rat S-9	23.3 + 3.8	34.2 + 5.9[d]	36.2 + 0.8[d]	28.0 + 1.7	27.3 + 3.9	34.5 +5.2[d]
Mouse mic.	34.9 + 3.8	41.1 + 5.2	53.0**	40.2 + 6.5	30.2 + 4.0	46.7 + 54.3[d,i]
Mouse S-9	31.7 + 4.9	34.0 + 3.7	40.6 + 3.1[e]	27.4 + 6.0	31.0**	—

a Mean percent of all metabolites as a function of total radioactivity $\pm$ SD; *n = 3, **n = 1.

b The reaction conditions are the same as described in Table 1.

c Significantly greater than corn oil, DBC, and PB at $p \leq 0.05$.

d Significantly greater than corn oil at $p \leq 0.05$.

e Significantly greater than DBA only at $p \leq 0.05$.

f Significantly greater than 3-MC rat S-9, mouse microsomes, and mouse S-9 at $p \leq 0.05$.

g Significantly greater than Aroclor rat S-9 at $p \leq 0.05$.

h Significantly greater than DBA rat S-9 and mouse S-9 at $p \leq 0.05$.

i Significantly greater than PB rat microsomes and rat S-9 at $p \leq 0.05$.

TABLE 6
Quantitation of Specific Metabolites of DBC Produced by Rat or Mouse Microsomes of S-9 Pretreated with 3-MC

| | % metabolite[a,b] | | | |
| | Rat | | Mouse | |
Metabolite	Microsomes	S-9	Microsomes	S-9
1-OH-DBC + minor				
2-OH-DBC	7.7 + 1.9[c]	3.1 + 1.2	5.8 + 1.1	4.1 + 1.7
3-OH-DBC	3.4 + 0.7[d]	3.9 + 1.2[d]	1.8 + 0.2	4.4 + 0.7[d]
5-OH-DBC	10.9 + 2.4[e]	1.2 + 0.0	2.9 + 1.4	1.7 + 0.1
6,6'-bis-(5-OH-DBC)	3.0 + 1.0[f]	0.6 + 0.1	2.4 + 0.4	0.9 + 0.3

[a] Mean percent of the specific metabolite as a function of total radioactivity ± SD, n = 3.

[b] The reaction conditions are the same as described in Table 1.

[c] Rat microsomes significantly greater than rat S-9 at $p \leq 0.05$.

[d] Rat microsomes and rat and mouse S-9 significantly greater than mouse microsomes at $p \leq 0.05$.

[e] Rat microsomes significantly greater than rat S-9, mouse microsomes, and mouse S-9 at $p \leq 0.05$.

[f] Rat microsomes significantly greater than rat S-9 and mouse S-9 at $p \leq 0.05$.

DBC comprised 2 to 8% of the total radioactivity, and the more polar unidentified metabolites of DBC accounted for 35% of the activity in the liver. After 48 h, over 50% of the total radioactivity was found in the feces.[63,64] In another study,[75] rats were exposed to ^{14}C-DBC by nose only for 60 min at concentrations of 1.4 and 13 µg/l of air. DBC was rapidly absorbed from the lung and translocated to other tissues such as the stomach, liver, and adrenals. Of the total radioactivity applied, 60 to 98% was eliminated from the body with half-times ranging from 1 to 16 h, and 95% was present in the feces. DBC was extensively metabolized before excretion; however, the metabolites were not identified. No glucuronide and sulfate components were detected in the excreted products.

In summary, for the metabolism of DBC both *in vitro* and *in vivo* in the rat and mouse, phenols, in particular the 5-OH and 3-OH, were the major products.

IV. *IN VITRO* MUTAGENICITY AND *IN VIVO* CARCINOGENESIS, INITIATION-PROMOTION, OF DBC AND DBA METABOLITES

In order to determine the metabolic sites responsible for activation, a number of studies have focused on DBC derivatives and DBC metabolites. With the addition of a methyl group at the seven position of DBC, the activity decreased significantly following mouse skin application[25] but not so if given subcutaneously.[68] The addition of an ethyl group at the seven position did not further decrease the activity.[26] In a rather complicated study, the administration of derivatives of DBC were given i.p. to induce hepatomas and subcutaneously to induce sarcomas. 5-Methyl, 6-methyl, 6,8-dimethyl, and N-acetyl DBC were active carcinogens following subcutaneous injection but were all negative in liver except N-acetyl when given i.p.[68] However, 3-methyl, 5,9-dimethyl, and 5,9-dimethyl-N-acetyl were active in liver when given i.p. but not in subcutaneous tissue. 5,9,N-trimethyl and 3,11-dimethyl were negative in both tissues. The 3-hydroxy, 3-acetoxy, and 3-methoxy were active in liver, similar to the methyl derivative, but not in subcutaneous tissue. 4-Methoxy and 4-acetoxy were active in both tissues, 5-hydroxy, 2-hydroxy, and 6-acetoxy were negative in both tissues, and 2- and 6-methoxy were active only in the subcutaneous tissue.[68] These data suggested that the five and seven positions and possibly the six position of DBC were involved in the sarcomagenic activity of DBC and the three and/or five and nine positions as well as the 3-hydroxy were involved in the hepatocarcinogenic activity of DBC. The four position and possibly the 4-hydroxy appeared to be involved in both tissues, whereas the 5-hydroxy, the 2-hydroxy, and the two position did not appear to be involved in either tissue.

Because of the difficulties in assessing *in vivo* carcinogenicity data, other approaches involving *in vitro* or short-term *in vivo* assays were used. Originally, DBC was found to be weakly mutagenic in tester strain TA98 with 10% Aroclor 1254 S9.[76] DBC was not mutagenic, however, in T98 and TA100 using a variety of S9 preparations from rat, mouse, and rabbit.[77] DBC was shown to be weakly mutagenic in a forward mutation assay in *Salmonella* strain TM677 using 8-azaguanine for selection.[77] On the other hand, in a cocultivation cell system using rat liver cells as the metabolizing layer and an epithelial cell line derived from embryonic hamster (DPI-3 cells) as the marker layer (mutation at the HGPRT locus was determined by resistance to 6-thioguanine toxicity), DBC was found to produce significantly higher rates of mutagenesis than BaP at concentrations of 0.4, 4.0, and 40.0 μM in the culture medium.[67] In similar studies using repair-deficient diploid human fibroblasts derived from a *Xeroderma pigmentosum* patient as the target cells and a human hepatoma cell line as a source for exogenous metabolism, DBC at twofold lower concentrations was more effective at inducing cytotoxicity and mutations in the target cells than 7-methyl DBC.[78]

For a series of DBC compounds, the cytosolic fraction was important in the mutagenicity of DBC, 3-methyl-DBC, and 5,9-dimethyl-DBC, all of which are potent hepatocarcinogens.[79] As mentioned previously, DBC-induced rat S9 DBC bacterial mutagenicity levels were a function of the amount of S9 as well as the inducer. In the cocultivation mutagenicity assay using rat liver and hamster epithelial cells, DBC produced significantly higher rates of mutagenesis than BaP, which was consistent with a higher rate of DBC metabolism relative to BaP. These data indicated that the cytosolic fraction was important in DBC metabolic activation.[79]

The DBC derivatives were tested for their mutagenicity in *Salmonella* assays and the mammalian cocultivation assay. In the forward mutation assay,[77] the data indicated that the activity of 3-OH, 4-OH, and 2-OH decreased in this order using 0.1 to 0.2 μg (0.37 to 0.74 nmol) per tube of compound at 10% 3-MC- or Aroclor 1254-induced S9 (10% represents the percentage of the total volume of 0.1 ml); 13c-OH and N-methyl DBC were not active. A HPLC fraction from the incubation of DBC with 3-MC-induced rat liver microsomes that cochromatographed with the 3-OH was mutagenic under the same conditions as the standard 3-OH DBC. In another study (unpublished), all available DBC metabolites (1-, 2-, 3-, 4-, 5-, 6-, and 13c-OH) were tested in the *Salmonella* reversion assay using TA98 and TA100 at 5 µg (18 nmol) per plate with and without 10% 3-MC-induced S9. DBC without activation appeared to be toxic. For TA98, 3-OH was mutagenic with S9. For TA100, 3-OH and 4-OH were mutagenic with S9. These data supported the idea that 3-OH and possibly 4-OH were mutagenic precursors of the ultimate metabolite(s). However, in the mammalian cocultivation assay,[67] 3-OH, 13c-OH, and *N*-methyl were mutagenic, while 2-OH and 4-OH were not active. The results of the latter study indicated that those metabolites inductively coupled to the nitrogen through resonance structures, that is, 3-OH, 13c-OH, and *N*-methyl were mutagenic and the nitrogen was involved in the metabolic activation of the parent compound through inductive mechanisms.

DBA and its metabolites were tested for their mutagenicity in *Salmonella* strains TA98 and TA100 with Aroclor 1254- or 3-MC-induced guinea-pig S9 fraction and in the mammalian V79 Chinese hamster lung cells with 3-MC-induced guinea pig S9 fraction.[80] DBA was found to be mutagenic over a dose range of 2 to 16 nmol per plate in the TA100 strain. Over this same dose range, 4-OH, 6-OH, 5,6-oxide, and N-oxide were not mutagenic in TA100. Of all the compounds tested that required guinea pig S9, including the 1,2-, 3,4-, and 5,6-dihydrodiol, the 3,4-dihydrodiol was the most mutagenic in the TA100 and V79 cells over similar dose ranges. In the TA98 strain, the 1,2-dihydrodiol was the most mutagenic. The most mutagenic compounds in both bacterial and V79 cells that did not require metabolic activation were the diol epoxides:

the *trans* or anti-3,4-dihydrodiol-1,2-epoxide was more active than the *cis* or *syn* form at similar dose ranges (2 to 16 nmol per plate for bacterial cells and 0.05 to 0.2 nmol per plate for mammalian cells). These data indicate that one active pathway for DBA was through the diol epoxide from the 3,4-dihydrodiol.[80] In another study (unpublished), in our laboratory, using the TA100 strain and the TA98 strain at the high-end dose of 5 µg (18 nmol) per plate with and without 3-MC-induced S9, DBA and its proximate metabolites were weakly to nonmutagenic. The metabolites included the 1,2, 3,4-, and 5,6-dihydrodiols, 5,6-oxide, and *N*-oxide. These latter results were consistent with the weak response of the TA100 strain and lack of response of the TA98 strain for DBA and its proximate metabolites using Aroclor 1254-induced rat S9.[80]

Our effort to determine the initiating ability of selected metabolites was based on short-term *in vivo* studies. We undertook an initiation-promotion study using 30 mice per group with an initiation dose of 200 nmol of the following metabolites in 50 µl of 95:5 acetone:DMSO: 1-OH, 2-OH, 3-OH, 4-OH, 5-OH, 6-OH of DBC; 5,6-oxide, *N*-oxide, and 5,6-dihydrodiol of DBA as well as DBC, DBA, and N-Me-DBC. No-treatment, solvent control, and TPA groups were also included. Two weeks after initiation, 2 µg of TPA was applied twice a week for 24 weeks. The data indicated that N-Me-DBC (20/28), DBC (25/29), and 4-OH (21/30) produced a significant number of animals with papillomas, and 2-OH (6/29), 6-OH (6/30), 3-OH (3/29), no initiation/TPA (2/29), 5-OH (1/29), and 1-OH (0/29) produced few animals with papillomas. The data for the initiating ability of DBC were consistent with the DNA binding in the skin for all compounds tested except for 6-OH and 3-OH DBC (reported below, where 3-OH showed the highest levels of binding in skin and 6-OH did not bind at all). One major difference in these studies was the use of the acetone-DMSO mix. All of the binding studies as well as the initiation-promotion and carcinogenicity studies involved only acetone as a solvent. From unpublished data we have shown that acetone will have the biggest impact on levels of DNA binding, that is, highest levels of binding. This would suggest that these studies need to be repeated with acetone as the solvent in order to compare the data from several studies.

With the DBA compounds, the data indicated that DBA (6/30), 5,6-oxide (4/29), N-oxide DBA (4/30), and 5,6-dihydrodiol DBA (4/29) produced few animals with papillomas. These data are consistent with the level of DNA binding for DBA. The 3,4-dihydrodiol of DBA was not available when these studies were done.

In order to address the differences seen between the initiating ability and the DNA binding results, the fact that two papillomas occurred in the TPA control group, and apparent effects of solvents, a smaller study with DBC and DBA, controls, and the 3,4-dihydrodiol of DBA and the 3-OH of DBC is being undertaken to resolve these differences.

In summary, these data indicated that the 3,4-dihydrodiol-1,2-epoxide of DBA was highly mutagenic relative to all other metabolites tested and that the 3,4-dihydrodiol appeared to be the proximate metabolite of DBA. On the other hand, for DBC it appeared that 3-OH and possibly 4-OH were the proximate metabolites based on the mutagenicity data.

V. DNA ADDUCTS

The formation of reactive metabolites, specifically DNA binding species, appears to be a critical step in the carcinogenicity of many chemical carcinogens.[81] Experimental evidence indicates that carcinogen-DNA adducts are associated with chromosome breakage and point mutations.[82–84] More recently, a prospective epidemiological study has shown that excretion of aflatoxin-DNA adducts was associated with an increased risk for hepatic cancer in a Chinese population.[85] Given this, it seemed plausible that the propensity of a compound to form DNA adducts was a reasonable first approximation of its carcinogenicity.

Therefore, the ability of DBC and DBA to form DNA adducts was investigated in some detail. Short-term DBC-DNA binding studies using radiolabeled DBC indicated that there was significant covalent reaction in vivo.[1,64] DBC, by any route of application, was found to form DNA adducts in the livers of mice at high levels, which corroborated the carcinogenicity studies detailed above.[47] As these data were refined using HPLC to resolve specific radioactive peaks in the DNA fractions, it became clear that the DBC-DNA interaction was more complex than that of compounds such as BaP, which appeared to form at least two discrete adduct regions by ^{32}P-postlabeling.[1,64,91] For example, Warshawsky et al. saw that there were two HPLC peaks, consistent with DBC-DNA binding.[64] This complexity was confirmed when more sensitive ^{32}P-postlabeling techniques were used to analyze DNA from animals treated with DBC. A total of at least seven discrete adduct zones could be identified from DBC-treated liver samples[86] (Figure 2). DBA appeared to be metabolized to DNA-binding species much less than DBC. Studies with radiolabeled compounds indicated that two adducts were formed.[87] This was corroborated by later studies utilizing ^{32}P-postlabeling to assay carcinogen-DNA adducts, as two radioactive spots were seen in DNA from DBA-treated skin samples[88–90] (Figure 3).

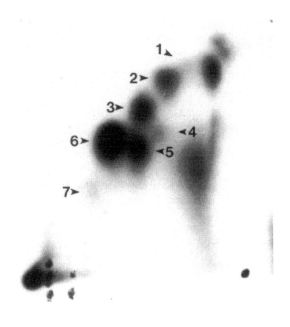

FIGURE 2. Typical autoradiogram of liver DNA of mice treated topically with DBC. Sample origin is at lower left corner. The number and arrows designate DBC treatment-related DNA adduct spots. Other radioactive areas are not treatment related, as they also appear in the untreated controls.[95]

Next, a series of studies were conducted to determine if the pattern of DNA adduction paralleled the target organs of these two compounds. Li et al.,[88] Roh et al.,[89] and Talaska et al.,[90] using a variety of sensitive ^{32}P-postlabeling methods, reported that DBA-DNA adducts formed predominately in the skin, with minor levels of adducts seen in the lung, but none at all in other tissues tested following topical application of DBA. This suggested that the binding of DBA to DNA followed the pattern of its carcinogenicity. Schurdak et al.[91] reported that the levels of DBC adducts were highest in the liver, skin, and lung of animals treated topically. This pattern of total binding could be altered somewhat by changing the route of administration. When DBC was administered by oral, i.p., or subcutaneous routes, the binding in tissues was liver >> kidney > lung > skin. These data indicated generally that those organs that were targets for

the carcinogenicity of these compounds were also the major targets for the production of DNA adducts.

There were distinct differences in the time courses of DBC- and DBA-DNA adducts in the skin following a single topical application of 100 µg (Figure 4). The levels at 24 h were approximately the same for both compounds. Somewhat surprisingly, the level of DBA-DNA adducts increased at 48 h to a level more than twice as high as that at 24 h. This was unusual when compared with DBC and many other carcinogens. The explanation for these data may at least partially be due to the fact that DBA was retained longer in the skin following application. Almost 40% of the total applied DBA was recovered from the skin at 48 h following treatment, while less than 20% of the applied DBC could be recovered from the skin at the same time.[64] Thus, it would seem that mouse skin specifically retained DBA at the site relative to DBC. DBC appeared to enter the systemic circulation faster due to the increased solubility of DBC, as evidenced by the high levels of hepatic DBC-DNA adducts. DBA-DNA adduct levels continued to increase linearly with time, suggesting that the parent compound was continually available to the activating metabolic enzymes in the skin.

In a comparison of DBC with BaP, blood protein and target organ DNA and protein binding were measured following topical application of DBC or BaP. This study sought to investigate factors that might account for differences in the DNA-binding activity between these compounds. Absorption of DBC from skin into blood and binding to blood proteins occurred linearly with dose. DBC bound to albumin at a 50-fold higher level than to globin, and levels of albumin adducts showed good correlation with levels of DNA adducts in liver. Hepatic preference over skin in DNA binding was found to be dose dependent. For

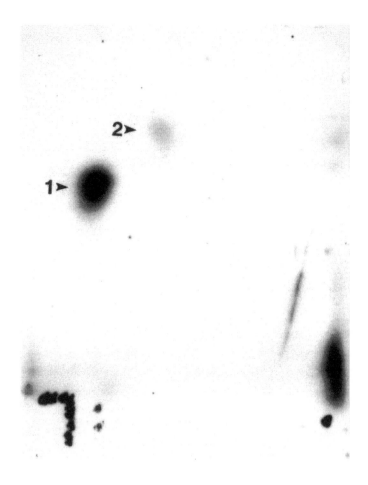

FIGURE 3. Typical autoradiogram of skin DNA in mice treated topically with DBA. Origins and markings are in Figure 2.[90]

comparison of [³H]BaP and [³H]DBC binding, doses of 1000 nmol per mouse were used, and the mice were sacrificed at 12, 24, and 48 h. The rate of DBC uptake from skin was 70% higher than for BaP over the first 24 h, which was reflected in 40 to 50% higher plasma levels of DBC. Skin protein and DNA binding were two- to fivefold higher for BP than DBC. Conversely, for DBC, total ³H levels in liver were two- to threefold higher, and liver DNA and protein binding were 15- to 20-fold and three- to fivefold higher, respectively. Blood protein adduct levels were similar for both chemicals, suggesting that the DBC metabolites formed in the liver were too reactive to reenter the systemic circulation.

These results indicated that more rapid absorption from skin and selective accumulation in the liver contribute to the greater liver DNA binding seen with DBC, but the types of liver metabolites appeared to be the major factor accounting for the binding difference.[92]

There appeared to be real qualitative differences in the initial products of metabolism between DBA and DBC. Using rat liver microsomes from 3-MC-pretreated rats, DBC[93] and DBA were metabolized to species that bound to DNA, RNA, and polynucleotides. The binding of DBC to poly-A, poly-U, and poly-C was significantly lower than to poly-G. DBC binding to nucleic acid was lower than for BaP

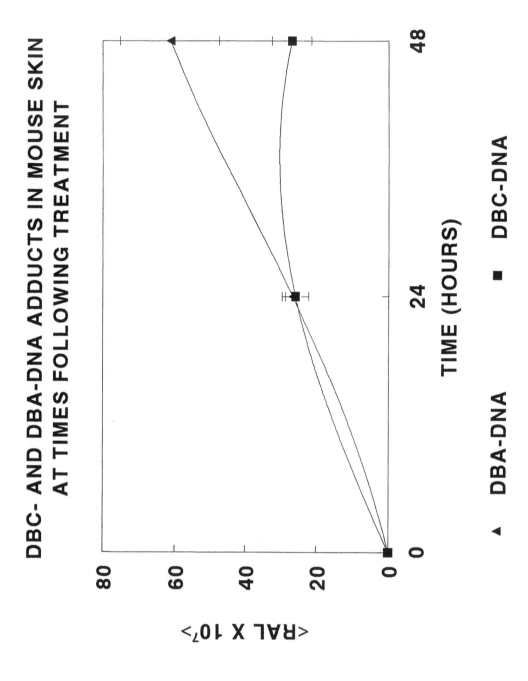

FIGURE 4. DBC and DBA-DNA adducts in mouse skin at times following topical treatment of 100 μg DBC or DBA to mice in 50 μl of acetone. The mice were sacrificed 24 h later, and DNA was isolated for adduct analysis using the ^{32}P-postlabeling technique.

(Table 7). When α-napthoflavone was added to the incubation mixture, the binding of DBC to poly-G was almost completely inhibited (Table 8). These results indicated that DBC-poly-G binding was dependent upon a microsomal hydroxylating enzyme system. The binding of DBC to poly-G was not affected by inhibitors or activators of epoxide hydrase, which suggested substitution,[93] not mediation via epoxide intermediates.

Following the digestion of nucleotides to nucleosides, HPLC and fluorescence spectroscopy studies, which were conducted using available standards, indicated that at least three different DBC-poly-G adducts were formed *in vitro*.[93] The fluorescence spectra of isolated adducts were red shifted, indicating that the π-electron system of DBC had not been disrupted by metabolism and subsequent binding, as this typically results in blue-shifted spectra. It was possible, however, that binding through the 3,4-epoxide may not have caused a significant blue shift because loss of the 1,2,3,4-ring altogether caused a very slight shift. The close resemblance of the adduct spectra with the N-methyl-DBC and the 4-OH-DBC suggested binding to poly-G through the 1,2,3,4-ring or through the nitrogen posi-

TABLE 7
Binding of DBC, DBA, and BaP to DNA, RNA, and Polynucleotides *In Vitro* in the Presence of a Rat Liver Microsomal Activating System[a]

	DBC[b]	DBA	BaP[b]
Calf thymus DNA	4.7 ± 8[c] (5)[d]	14.7 ± 5.1 (4)	55.5 ± 1.8 (3)[f]
Yeast RNA	3.9 ± 0.2 (3)	23.7 ± 9.9 (4)	15.1 ± 0.3 (3)
Poly [G]	13.6 ± 0.5 (3)[g]	78.3 ± 13.8 (4)[h]	122.5 ± 4.1 (3)[e,i]
Poly [A]	2.1 ± 0.7 (5)	9.3 ± 2.0 (4)	10.2 ± 0.9 (5)
Poly [U]	2.8 ± 0.8 (5)	13.0 ± 2.8 (4)	7.8 ± 0.6 (3)
Poly [C]	1.2 ± 0.2 (3)	5.2 ± 1.7 (4)	4.3 ± 0.2 (3)

[a] 3-Methylcholanthrene-induced microsomal preparations prepared from male Sprague-Dawley rats incubated with 2 μmol of nucleic acid and 6 nmol of DBC, DBA, or BaP.

[b] From Reference 93.

[c] pmol DBC, DBA, or BaP bound/μmol DNA, RNA, or polynucleotide mean ± SD.

[d] Number of determinations.

[e] Significantly greater than all other BaP-binding data at $p \leq 0.05$.

[f] Significantly greater than BaP-RNA binding at $p \leq 0.05$.

[g] Significantly greater than all other DBC-binding data at $p \leq 0.05$.

[h] Significantly greater than all other DBA-binding data at $p \leq 0.05$.

[i] Significantly greater than all other binding data at $p \leq 0.05$.

TABLE 8

Effect of Modifiers of Rat Microsomal Enzyme Activity on DBC and DBA Binding to Poly-G[a]

		Binding as % of control	
Modifier	Concentration	DBC[b]	DBA
α-Napthoflavone	10^{-3} M	2.7 ± 3.0 (3)[c,d]	2.5 ± 1.8[d] (4)
	10^{-4} M	4.5 ± 7.6 (3)[d]	17.6 ± 4.7[d] (4)
Trichloropropene oxide	10^{-3} M	82 ± 16 (2)	199 ± 30 (4)
	10^{-4} M	84 ± 13 (2)	249 ± 30 (4)
Cyclohexene oxide	10^{-3} M	98 ± 16 (3)	196 ± 22 (4)
	10^{-4} M	107 ± 11 (3)	129 ± 22 (4)
Styrene oxide	10^{-3} M	94 ± 10 (2)	197 ± 45 (4)
	10^{-4} M	92 ± 13 (2)	103 ± 18 (4)

[a] The incubation mixture as described in Table 7, with the addition of the modifier at two different concentrations.

[b] From Reference 93.

[c] Number of determinations; mean ± SD.

[d] Significantly less than all other modifiers at $p \leq 0.05$.

tion of DBC. The adduct spectra were consistent with the notion that binding through one of these positions was preceded by metabolism at another site, as indicated by *in vivo* ^{32}P-postlabeling studies and mutagenicity data.

The highest DBA-nucleic acid binding was to poly-G (Table 7); however, this was at lower levels than BaP. α-Naphthoflavone inhibited DBA poly-G binding almost completely, while styrene oxide, cyclohexene oxide, and trichloropropene oxide (TCPO) increased poly-G binding relative to control binding (Table 8). These results indicated that DBA-poly-G binding was dependent upon a microsomal hydroxylating enzyme system, and the observed increase in binding was attributed to the accumulation of epoxide intermediates that react with nucleic acids. This indicated that the types of metabolites involved in binding are similar for BaP and DBA. Similar procedures, as described above, were being used to look at the adducts of DBA with poly G, and so far, the data have indicated two HPLC peaks. The fluorescence spectra of these peaks indicated two polar adducts that are blue shifted from DBA and that the peak at 25 min was indicative of binding through the 3,4-position of DBA, similar to the 3,4-dihydrodiol.

These data suggested that while P450 enzymes were essential to the formation of DNA-binding species for both compounds, dihydrodiol formation was more important for DBA. This supposition was corroborated by data indicating that the major metabolites of DBA were the corresponding 1,2-, 3,4-, and 5,6-dihydrodiols, while those of DBC were the 3-, 5-, 4-, 6-, and 2-phenols. These metabolites were applied to mouse skin and the resulting carcinogen-DNA adducts analyzed. Schurdak et al. reported that 3-OH-DBC appeared to be the proximate genotoxin in the liver, as application of this metabolite produced adducts identical to those when the parent compound was applied.[94] In the skin, 3-OH-DBC produced a different spectrum of adducts, including several not observed with the parent material. These studies were extended to show that there was substantial agreement with the proportions of different adducts produced in the liver with either DBC or 3-OH-DBC, but that the latter compound altered the spectrum of DBC-DNA adducts in both skin and lung.[95] In addition, several other metabolites were applied and found to radically alter the pattern of DNA binding seen with DBC. For example, the 1-, 5-, 6-, and 13c-OH DBC metabolites did not produce treatment-related adducts in skin, liver, or lung. 4-OH-DBC produced adducts in all three tissues; however, these were substantially different than those obtained for DBC. Shurdak et al. were also the first to show that methylation of the nitrogen of DBC reduced the hepatic levels of DBC-DNA adducts drastically, while producing approximately the same level of adducts in the skin.[96] In this regard, it was interesting that N-methyl-DBC was a skin carcinogen of about equal potency as DBC, while it did not produce tumors in the liver. Finally, it was shown that N-methyl-DBC greatly altered the DBC-DNA adduct pattern in the skin, so it appeared that, although different adducts were produced, they were about equally genotoxic in this tissue.[25,71]

Roh et al.[89] and Talaska et al.[90] reported that a metabolite, DBA-3,4-dihydrodiol, formed higher levels of DBA-DNA adducts than did the parent compound, suggesting that this compound was in the pathway of DBA activation. This result was consistent with earlier reports of the mutagenic activities of DBA metabolites.[80] Interestingly, when DBA-5,6-dihydrodiol was applied

topically, two different treatment-related adducts were observed. These adducts were not seen when DBA was applied; however, very low levels were seen when samples obtained from DBA-3,4-dihydrodiol-treated animals were analyzed using ultrasensitive assay conditions. However, when DBA-3,4-dihydrodiol was applied and analyzed using nuclease P_1, all four adducts could be detected. These results suggested that the major route of DBA activation to DNA binding in skin was through the formation of DBA-3,4-dihydrodiol and subsequent metabolism to a diolepoxide and a minor pathway that proceeded through a bis-dihydrodiol epoxide.[90]

In summary, the levels of DBA- and DBC-DNA adducts have proven consistent with the target organ carcinogenic activity of DBC, DBA, and their metabolites.[97] This relationship appeared to be both qualitative and quantitative. The hepatic carcinogenicity of DBC was associated with high levels of all adducts, with those with higher polarity predominating (i.e., adduct 6). In the skin, also a target organ, adducts with lower affinity for the stationary phase were more commonly seen (i.e., adducts 2 and 3). A comparison of DNA adducts with the preliminary skin carcinogenicity data (initiation-promotion studies treated with the same doses of DBC or its metabolites) indicated that nonpolar adducts 1 and 2 were associated with skin carcinogenicity. These adducts could explain 97% of the variation in dermal carcinogenicity, whereas adducts with higher polarity (6 and 7) correlated with carcinogenicity to a much lesser extent, and adduct 3 not at all.[95] A recent study showed that a single i.p. injection of DBC produced tumors in the lung at high frequency in a sensitive strain of mouse.[49] DBC-DNA adduct 3 accounted for over 60% of the total adducts in the lung, and while this adduct did not appear to be related to tumors in the skin, initial analysis suggested that this adduct was responsible for the lung tumors in the A/J mouse strain.

A recent report indicated that mouse mitochondial DNA, as well as nuclear DNA, could be a major target for DBC and its hepatocarcinogenic alkylated derivatives. These data support the hypothesis that carcinogen-induced DNA damage in mitochondrial as well as nuclear may play a role in one or more steps of carcinogenesis.[98] Finally, recent evidence indicated that both DBC and DBA induce micronuclei in cultured human lympocytes.[99] DBC produced a significant increase above background, but the dose response tended to plateau above 0.1 µg/ml, whereas DBC showed an effect only at high doses above controls at 5 and 10 µg/ml. These data indicated that the micronucleus assay would be another overall sensitive endpoint for measuring N-heterocyclic compounds. It has been shown in mouse skin keratinocytes that there is a strong correlation between DNA adducts and micronuclei induction for DBC, and that the combination of adduct 3 and adduct 6 levels correlated better with micronuclei induction than total adduct levels.[100] This would indicate that specific adducts may be better predictors of genotoxicity than combined adduct levels and would be consistent with target organ specificity.

Although it appeared for total levels of DNA adduction, there was a clear correspondence between adduct levels, target organ activity, and carcinogenicity for DBC on the gross level; particular adducts and effects remained enigmatic. Different patterns of adducts were seen in different target tissues. The differences in adduct formation in these organs were likely due to tissue-specific activities of metabolic enzymes; nonetheless, adducts in each target tissue appeared to induce tumors. Progress on the chemical identification of the adducts is underway using a variety of *in vitro* and *in vivo* techniques to resolve some of the critical questions.

VI. SUMMARY

In summary, DBC is a potent liver, lung, and skin carcinogen in mouse by both local and systemic administration. It is also a carcinogen in the dog, rat, and hamster. DBA, on the other hand, is a skin and lung carcinogen in the mouse. DBC is metabolized to phenols, with the 3- and 4-OH being the possible proximate carcinogenic metabolites of DBC. DBC forms at least seven adducts in the target tissues, and the major adduct in the lung correlates with the K-*ras* mutations in the lung. The major mutation in the lung is on the third base of the 61st codon, which was seen for the first time in chemically induced lung tumors in the mouse. The major adduct pattern is different in each target tissue, which suggests a different activation mechanism in each tissue (Table 9). The major pathway for DBC is not well resolved at this point, but data suggest that both two- and one-electron oxidation pathways may be involved[101] (Figure 5). DBA is metabolized to dihydrodiols, phenols, and oxides. The proximate carcinogenic metabolite appears to be the 3,4-dihydrodiol. Only two major adducts appear to be formed in the skin with two minor adducts. These data suggest that the major pathway involves diol epoxides and that the minor pathway involves *bis*-dihydrodiol epoxides (Figure 6). Work is in progress to determine the chemical structures of the adducts, to resolve the questions concerning the activation pathways for both DBC and DBA in liver and skin, and to determine the mutations produced in ras and p53 genes associated with the target tissues. Finally, it will be important to correlate specific adducts with specific mutations and to determine the rela-

TABLE 9

Comparison of DBC and DBA Activation in Hsd:ICR(Br) Mouse

Test compound		Total DNA adduct formation			
		Total[b]	Major adducts[c]	Tumor formation	
DBC	Liver	123.0	6 > 5	37/50[d]	
	Lung	5.4	3 > 6		
	Skin	18.3	2, 3	42/50[d]	26/30[e]
3-OH-DBC[a]	Liver	428.4	6 > 5		
	Lung	19.8	6 > 3, 2		
	Skin	33.2	3		
DBA	Skin	5.0	1, 2	27/50[d]	17/30[e]
3,4-Dihydrodiol[a]	Skin	9.6	1, 2		
5,6-Dihydrodiol[a]	Skin	3.6	3, 4		

[a] Major metabolites.[45,52,53,65,67,72,73]

[b] 100-μg dose of parent compound or metabolite — relative adduct labeling x 10^7 under carrier-free conditions.[90,95]

[c] Major adduct assignments: DBC, total of seven adducts; DBA, total of two adducts.[90,95]

[d] Carcinogenesis protocol: 50 nmol twice weekly; Hsd:ICR(Br).[47]

[e] Initiation/promotion protocol. 200 nmol once, followed 2 weeks later by 2 μg of TPA twice weekly; Hsd:ICR(Br).[48]

tionship between DNA repair of these adducts and p53 as well as the effects of DBC and DBA on RNA and protein.

ACKNOWLEDGMENTS

We thank Leva Wilson for preparing this manuscript. Work reported in this review was supported in part by NIEHS ES-04203-07, USEPA R818088, NCI-CA23515, DOE DEACO2-82ER60076, and NIEHS 5P 30ES06096 and P42 ES04908. This work represents the research input of the following people from this laboratory: graduate students David B. Stong (NIOSH OH1701 and NIEHS training grant ES0703), Bernadette Lindquist (NIEHS 03409 and Ryan Foundation Fellowship), Liping Wan, John Meier, and Suresh Krishnan (NIOSH OH022880 and P42 ES04908); postdoctoral students Jeffry Dietz (NIEHS Training Grant ES-07250), Susan Fremont, and Patrick O'Connor (NIEHS Training Grant ES07278); faculty members Jaehoon Roh (Visiting Professor from Seoul, Korea), William Barkley, Rita Schoeny, Marian Miller, and Gordon Livingston; staff members Raymond Reilman, Marlene Schamer, Kathy LaDow, Andrea Andringa, Tyrone Collins, Lois Hollingsworth, Betty Myers, and Betty Ann Smiddy; and collaborators Gary Stoner of Ohio State University and Mark Schurdak and Kurt Randerath of Baylor College of Medicine.

242

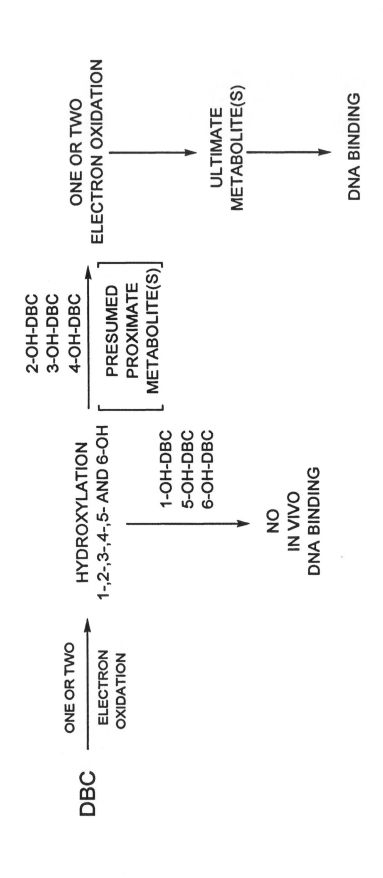

FIGURE 5. DBC metabolic activation pathway.

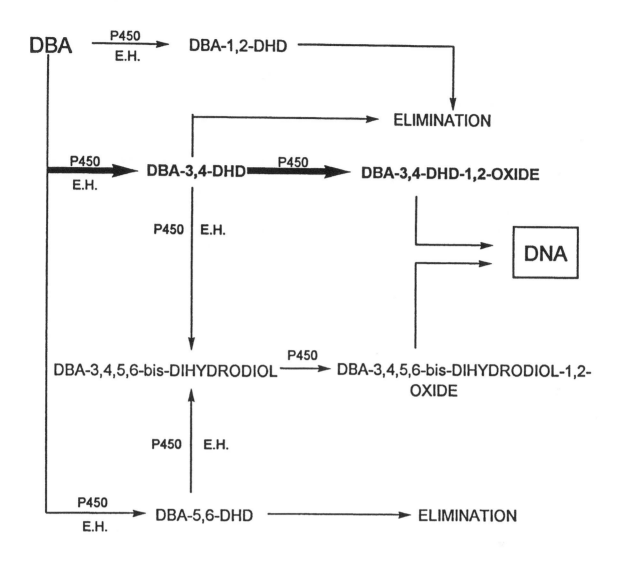

FIGURE 6. DBA metabolic activation pathway.

REFERENCES

1. **Warshawsky, D.,** Environmental sources, carcinogencity, mutagenicity, metabolism and DNA binding of nitrogen and sulfur heterocyclic aromatics, *Environ. Carcinogen. Ecotoxicol. Rev.*, 10, 1, 1992.

2. **Warshawsky, D., Barkley, W., and Bingham, E.,** Factors affecting carcinogenic potential of mixtures, *Fundam. Appl. Toxicol.*, 20, 376, 1993.

3. **Bingham, E., Trosset, R., and Warshawsky, D.,** Carcinogenic potential of petroleum hydrocarbons, *J. Environ. Pathol. Toxicol.*, 3, 483, 1979.

4. **Trosset, R. P., Warshawsky, D., Menefee, C., and Bingham, E.,** Investigation of Selected Potential Environmental Contaminants: Asphalts and Coal Tar Pitch, Publ. Environmental Protection Agency, 56012-77-005, 1978.

5. **IARC,** Monographs on the Evaluation of the Carcinogenic Risk of Chemicals to Humans, Vol. 33, Polynuclear Aromatic Compounds, Part 2, Carbon Blacks, Mineral Oils and Some Nitroarenes, International Agency for Research into Cancer, Lyon, France, 1984.

6. **IARC,** Monographs on the Evaluation of the Carcinogenic Risk of Chemicals to Hu-

mans, Vol. 34, Polynuclear Aromatic Compounds, Part 3, Industrial Exposures in Aluminium Production, Coal Gasification, Coke Production and Iron Steel Founding, International Agency for Research into Cancer, Lyon, France, 1984.

7. **IARC,** Monographs on the Evaluation of the Carcinogenic Risk of Chemicals to Humans, Vol. 35, Polynuclear Aromatic Compounds, Part 4, Bitumens, Coal-tars and Derived Products, Shale-Oils and Soots, International Agency for Research into Cancer, Lyon, France, 1985.

8. **IARC,** Monographs on the Evaluation of Carcinogenic Risk of the Chemical to Man, Vol. 3, Certain Polycyclic Aromatic Hydrocarbons and Heterocyclic Compounds, International Agency for Research into Cancer, Lyon, France, 1973.

9. **IARC,** Monographs on the Evaluation of the Carcinogenic Risk of Chemicals to Humans, Vol. 32, Polynuclear Aromatic Compounds, Part 1, Chemical, Environmental and Experimental Data, International Agency for Research into Cancer, Lyon, France, 1983.

10. **Santodonato, J., Howard, P., and Basu, D.,** Health and ecological assessment of polynuclear aromatic hydrocarbons, *J. Environ. Pathol. Toxicol.*, 5, 1, 1981.

11. **Sawicki, E., Meeker, J. E., and Morgan, M.,** Polynuclear aza compounds in automotive exhaust, *Arch. Environ. Health*, 11, 773, 1965.

12. **Sawicki, E., Meeker, J. E., and Morgan, M.,** The quantitative composition of air pollution source effluents in terms of aza heterocyclic compounds and polynuclear aromatic hydrocarbons, *Int. J. Air Water Pollut.*, 9, 291, 1965.

13. **White, L. D.,** Collection, Separation, Identification and Quantitation of Selected PAHs and Metals in Coal Tar and Coke Oven Emissions, Ph.D. thesis, University of Cincinnati, 1975.

14. **Wright, C. W., Later, D. W., Pelroy, R. A., Mahlum, D. D., and Wilson, B. W.,** Comparative chemical and biological analysis of coal tar-based therapeutic agents to other

coal-derived materials, *J. Appl. Toxicol.*, 5, 80, 1985.

15. **Van Duuren, G. L., Bilbao, J. A., and Joseph, C. A.,** The carcinogenic nitrogen heterocyclics in cigarette-smoke condensate, *J. Natl. Cancer Inst.*, 25, 53, 1960.

16. **Serth, R. W. and Hughes, T. W.,** Polycyclic organic matter and trace element contents of carbon black vent gas, *Environ. Sci. Technol.*, 14, 298, 1980.

17. **Ho, C., Clark, B. R., Guerin, M. R., Barkenbus, B. D., and Rao, E. J. L.,** Analytical and biological analyses of test materials form the synthetic fuel technologies. IV. Studies of chemical structure-mutagenic activity relationships of aromatic nitrogen compounds relevant to synfuels, *Mutat. Res.*, 85, 335, 1981.

18. **Shinohara, R., Kido, A., Okamoto, Y., and Takeshita, R.,** Determination of trace azaarenes in water by gas chromatography and gas chromatography mass spectrometry, *J. Chromatogr.*, 256, 81, 1983.

19. **Ciccioli, P., Brancaleoni, E., Cecinato, A., DiPalo, C., Buttini, P., and Liberti, A.,** Fractionation of polar polynuclear aromatic hydrocarbons present in industrial emissions and atmospheric samples and their determination by gas chromatography-mass spectrometry, *J. Chromatogr.*, 351, 451, 1986.

20. **Cautreels, W. and Van Cauwenberghe, K.,** Determination of organic compounds in airborne particulate matter by gas chromatography mass spectrometry, *Atmos. Environ.*, 10, 447, 1976.

21. **Warshawsky, D.,** unpublished data.

22. **Armstrong, E. C. and Bonser, G. M.,** Squamous carcinoma of the forestomach and other lesions in mice following oral administration of 3,4,5,6-dibenzcarbazole, *Br. J. Cancer*, 4, 203, 1950.

23. **Boyland, E. and Brues, A. M.,** The carcinogenic action of dibenzcarbazoles, *Proc. R. Soc. London, Ser. B*, 122, 429, 1937.

24. **Strong, L. C., Smith, G. M., and Gardner, W. J.,** Induction of tumors by 3,4,5,6-

244

dibenzcarbazole in male mice of the CBA strain, which develops spontaneous hepatoma, *Yale J. Biol. Med.*, 10, 335, 1938.

25. **Kirby, A. H. M. and Peacock, P. R.,** The influence of methylation on carcinogenic activity. I. *N*-methyl-3,4,5,6-dibenzcarbazole, *Brit. J. Exp. Pathol.*, 27, 179, 1946.

26. **Kirby, A. H. M.,** The carcinogenic activity of *N*-ethyl-3,4,5,6-dibenzcarbazole. *Biochem. J.*, 1, 42, 1948.

27. **Bonser, G. M., Clayson, D. B., Jull, J. W., and Pyrah, L. N.,** The carcinogenic properties of 2-amino-1-naphthol hydrochloride and its parent amine 2-naphthylamine, *Br. J. Cancer*, 6, 412, 1954.

28. **Buu-Hoi, N. P.,** New developments in chemical carcinogenesis by polycyclic hydrocarbons and related heterocycles: a review, *Cancer Res.*, 24, 1511, 1964.

29. **Lacassagne, A., Buu-Hoi, N., Zajdela, F., and Xuong, N. D.,** Relations entre la structure moleculaire et l'activite cancerogene dans la serie du carbazole, *Bull. Cancer*, 42, 1, 1955.

30. **Andervont, H. G. and Edwards, J. E.,** Hepatic changes and subcutaneous and pulmonary tumors induced by subcutaneous injection of 3,4,5,6-dibenzcarbazole, *JNCI*, 2, 139, 1941.

31. **Andervont, H. B. and Shimkin, M. R.,** Biological testing of carcinogens. II. Pulmonary-tumor-induction technique, *JNCI*, 1, 225, 1940.

32. **Boyland, E. and Mawson, E. H.,** Changes in the liver of mice after administration of 3,4,5,6-dibenzcarbazole, *Biochem. J.*, 32, 1460, 1938.

33. **Bonser, G. M., Crabbe, J. G. S., Jull, J. W., and Pyrah, L. N.,** Induction of epithelial neoplasms in the urinary bladder of the dog by intravesical injection of a chemical carcinogen, *J. Pathol. Bacteriol.*, 68, 561, 1954.

34. **Sellakumar, A. and Shubik, P.,** Carcinogenicity of 7H-dibenzo[*c,g*]carbazole in the respiratory tract of hamsters, *J. Natl. Cancer Inst.*, 48, 1641, 1972.

35. **Nagel, D. L., Stenback, F., Clayson, D. B., and Wallcave, L.,** Intratracheal instillation studies with 7H-dibenzo[*c,g*]carbazole in the Syrian hamster, *J. Natl. Cancer Inst.*, 57, 119, 1976.

36. **Sellakumar, A. R., Stenback, F., Rowland, J., and Shubik, P.,** Tumor induction by 7H-dibenzo[*c,g*]carbazole in the respiratory tract of Syrian hamsters, *J. Toxicol. Environ. Health*, 3, 935, 1977.

37. **Montesano, R., Saffiotti, U., and Shubik, P.,** The role of topical and systemic factors in experimental respiratory carcinogenesis, in Hanna, M. G., Nettesheim, P., and Gilbert, J. R., Eds., *Inhalation Carcinogenesis*, U.S. Atomic Energy Commission Symposium Series No. 18, 1970, 353.

38. **Badger, G. M., Cook, J. W., Hewett, C. L., Kennaway, E. L., Kennaway, N. M., Martin, R. H., and Robinson, A. M.,** The production of cancer by pure hydrocarbons. V. *Proc. R. Soc. London Ser. B*, 129, 439, 1940.

39. **Barry, G., Cook, J. W., Haslewood, G. A. D., Hewett, C. L., Hieger, I., and Kennaway, E. L.,** The production of cancer by pure hydrocarbons. III. *Proc. R. Soc. London, Ser. B*, 117, 318, 1935.

40. **Lacassagne, A., Buu-Hoi, N. P., Zajdela, F., Royer, R., and Hubert-Habart, M.,** Activite cancerogene des dibenzacridines bisangulaires, *Bull. Cancer*, 42, 186, 1955.

41. **Bachmann, W. E., Cook, J. W., Dansi, A., de Worms, C. G. M., Haslewood, G. A. D., Hewett, C .L., and Robinson, A. M.,** The production of cancer by pure hydrocarbons. IV. *Proc. R. Soc. London Ser. B*, 123, 343, 1937.

42. **Wynder, E. L. and Hoffman, D.,** Ein experimenteller Beitrag zur Tabakrauchkanzerogenese, *Dtsch. Med. Wochenschr.*, 25, 53, 1963.

43. **Deutsch-Wenzel, R. P., Brune, H., and Grimmer, G.,** Experimental studies on the carcinogenicity of five nitrogen containing polycyclic aromatic compounds directly injected into rat lungs, *Cancer Lett.*, 20, 97, 1983.

44. **Stenbaeck, F. and Rowland, J.,** Experimental respiratory carcinogenesis in hamsters: environmental, physicochemical and biological aspects, *Oncology*, 36, 63, 1979.

45. **Wan, L., Xue, W., Schneider, J., Reilman, R., Radike, M., and Warshawsky, D.,** Comparative metabolism of 7H-dibenzo[*c,g*]carbazole and dibenz[*a,j*]acridine by mouse and rat liver microsomes, *Chem. Biol. Interact.*, 81, 131, 1992.

46. **Warshawsky, D. and Barkley, W.,** Comparative carcinogenic potencies of 7H-dibenzo[*c,g*]carbazole, dibenz[*a,j*]acridine and benzo[*a*]pyrene in mouse skin, *Cancer Lett.*, 37, 337, 1987.

47. **Warshawsky, D., Barkley, W., Miller, M. L., LaDow, K., and Andringa, A.,** Carcinogenicity of 7H-dibenzo[*c,g*]carbazole, dibenz[*a,j*]acridine and benzo[*a*]pyrene in mouse skin and liver following topical application, *Toxicology*, 9, 135, 1994.

48. **Warshawsky, D., Barkley, W., Miller, M. L., LaDow, K., and Andringa, A.,** Comparative tumor-initiating ability of 7H-dibenzo[*c,g*]carbazole and dibenz[*a,j*]acridine in mouse skin, *Toxicology*, 71, 233, 1992.

49. **Warshawsky, D., Talaska, G., Schamer, M., Collins, T., Galati, A., You, L., and Stoner, G.,** Carcinogenicity, DNA adduct formation and K-ras activation by 7H-dibenzo[*c,g*]carbazole in strain A mouse lung, *Carcinogenesis*, in press.

50. **Warshawsky, D., Hollingsworth, L., Reilman, R., and Stong, D. B.,** The metabolism of dibenz[*a,j*]acridine in the isolated perfused lung, *Cancer Lett.*, 28, 317, 1985.

51. **Rosario, C. A., Holder, G. M., and Duke, C. C.,** Synthesis of potential metabolites of dibenz[*a,j*]acridine: phenols and dihydrodiols, *J. Org. Chem.*, 52, 1064, 1987.

52. **Gill, G. H., Duke, C. C., Rosario, C. A., Ryan, A. J., and Holder, G. M.,** Dibenz[*a,j*]acridine metabolism: identification of *in vitro* products formed by liver microsomes from 3-methylcholanthrene pretreated rats, *Carcinogenesis*, 7, 1371, 1986.

53. **Schneider, J., Xue, W., and Warshawsky, D.,** Fluorescence spectroscopic studies on the identification and quantitation of metabolites of 7H-dibenzo[*c,g*]carbazole and dibenz[*a,j*]acridine, *Chem. Biol. Interact.*, 93, 139, 1994.

54. **Gill, G. H., Duke, C. C., Ryan, A. J., and Holder, G. M.,** Dibenz[*a,j*]acridine: distribution of metabolites formed by liver and lung microsomes from control and pretreated rats, *Carcinogenesis*, 8, 425, 1987.

55. **Thakker, D. R., Shirai, N., Levin, W., Ryan, D. E., Thomas, P. E., Lehr, R. E., Conney, A. H., and Jerina, D. M.,** Metabolism of dibenz(*c,h*)acridine by rat liver enzymes and by cytochrome P450c with and without added epoxide hydrase, *Proc. Annu. Meet., Am. Assoc. Cancer Res.*, 26, A114, 1985.

56. **Sayer, J. M., Lehr, R. E., Kumar, S., Yagi, K., Yeh, H. J. C., Holder, G. M., Duke, C. C., Silverton, J. V., Gibson, C., and Jerina, D. M.,** Comparative solvolytic reactivity of bay-region diol-epoxide derived from dibenz[*a,j*]anthracene and dibenzacridine, *J. Am. Chem. Soc.*, 112, 1177, 1990.

57. **Sugiyanto, C., Scharping, M. E., McManus, M. E., Birkett, D. J., Holder, G. M., and Ryan, A. J.,** The formation of proximate carcinogens from three polycyclic aromatic compounds by human liver microsomes, *Xenobiotica*, 22, 1299, 1992.

58. **Roberts-Thomson, S. J., McManus, M. E., Tukey, R. H., Gonzalez, F. J., and Holder, G. M.,** Metabolism of polycyclic aza-aromatic carcinogens catalyzed by four expressed human cytochromes P450, *Cancer Res.*, 55, 1052, 1995.

59. **Nelson, D. R., Kamataki, T., Waxman, D. J., Guengerich, F. P., Estabrook, R. W., Reyereisen, R., Gonzalez, F. J., Coon, M. J., Gunsalus, I. C., Gotoh, O., Okuda, K., and Nebert, D. W.,** The P450 superfamily: update on new sequences, gene mapping, accession numbers, early trivial names of enzymes and nomenclature, *DNA Cell Biol.*, 12, 1, 1993.

60. **Okey, A. B.,** Enzyme induction in the cytochrome P450 system, *Pharm. Ther.*, 45, 241, 1990.

61. **Duke, C. C., Holder, G. M., Rosario, C. A., and Ryan, A. J.,** Stereochemistry of the major rodent liver microsomal metabolites of the carcinogen dibenz[*a,j*]acridine, *Chem. Res. Toxicol.*, 1, 294, 1988.

62. **Warshawsky, D., Hollingsowth, L., Stong, D. B., and Smiddy, B. A.,** Pulmonary metabolism of dibenz[*a,j*]acridine, in *PAHs: Chemistry, Characterization and Carcinogenesis*, Cooke, M. and Dannis, A., Eds., Battelle Press, Columbus, OH, 1986, 961.

63. **Robinson, H. K., Duke, C. C., Holder, G. M., and Ryan, A. J.,** The metabolism of the carcinogen dibenz[*a,j*]acridine in isolated rat hepatocyte and *in vivo* in rats, *Xenobiotica*, 20, 457, 1990.

64. **Warshawsky, D., Dietz, J. J., Reilman, R., Xue, W., LaDow, K., Roh, J., and Talaska, G.,** Disposition of 7H-dibenzo[*c,g*]carbazole and dibenz[*a,j*]acridine in the mouse following topical application, *Polycyclic Aromatic Hydrocarbons*, 3 (Suppl.), 711, 1993.

65. **Perin, F., Dufour, M., Mispelter, J., Ekert, B., Kunneke, C., Oesch, F., and Zajdela, F.,** Heterocyclic polycyclic aromatic hydrocarbon carcinogenesis: 7H-dibenzo[*c,g*]carbazole metabolism by microsomal enzymes from mouse and rat liver, *Chem. Biol. Interact.*, 35, 267, 1981.

66. **Warshawsky, D. and Meyer, B. L.,** The metabolism of 7H-dibenzo[*c,g*]carbazole, a *N*-heterocyclic aromatic in the isolated perfused lung, *Cancer Lett.*, 12, 153, 1981.

67. **Stong, D. B., Christian, R. T., Jayasimhulu, K., Wilson, R. M., and Warshawsky, D.,** The chemistry and biology of 7H-dibenzo[*c,g*]carbazole: synthesis and characterization of selected derivatives, metabolism in rat liver preparations and mutagenesis mediated by cultured rat hepatocytes, *Carcinogenesis*, 10, 419, 1989.

68. **Szafarz, D., Perin, F., Valero, D., and Zajdela, F.,** Structure and carcinogenicity of dibenzo[*c,g*]carbazole derivatives, *Biosci. Rep.*, 8, 633, 1988.

69. **Kato, R.,** Metabolic activation of mutagenic heterocyclic aromatic amines from protein pyrolysates, *CRC Crit. Rev. Toxicol.*, 16, 307, 1986.

70. **Schut, H. A. J.,** Metabolism of carcinogenic amino derivatives in various species and DNA alkylation by their metabolites, *Drug Metab. Rev.*, 15, 753, 1984.

71. **Perin, F., Valero, D., Mispelter, J., and Zajdela, F.,** *In vitro* metabolism of *N*-methyl-dibenzo[*c,g*]carbazole, a potent sarcomatogen devoid of hepatotoxic and hepatocarcinogenic properties, *Chem. Biol. Interact.*, 48, 281, 1984.

72. **Xue, W. and Warshawsky, D.,** Synthesis and characterization of monohydroxylated derivatives of 7H-dibenzo[*c,g*]carbazole, *Chem. Res. Toxicol.*, 5, 130, 1992.

73. **Xue, W., Schneider, J., Jayasimhulu, K., and Warshawsky, D.,** Acetylation of phenolic derivatives of 7H-dibenzo[*c,g*]carbazole: identification and quantitation of major metabolites by rat liver microsomes, *Chem. Res. Toxicol.*, 6, 345, 1993.

74. **Warshawsky, D., Schamer, M., Schneider, J., Xue, W., Reilman, R., and Talaska, G.,** Characterization of 7H-dibenzo[*c,g*]carbazole-DNA adducts in the mouse following topical application, *Proc. Annu. Meet., Am. Assoc. Cancer Res.*, 33, A825, 1992.

75. **Bond, J. A., Ayres, P. H., Medinsky, M. A., Cheng, Y. S., Hirshfield, D., and McClellan, R. O.,** Disposition and metabolism of [^{14}C] dibenzo[*c,g*]-carbazole aerosols in rats after inhalation, *Fundam. Appl. Toxicol.*, 7, 76, 1986.

76. **Salamone, M. F., Heddle, J. A., and Katz, M.,** The mutagenic activity of thirty polycyclic aromatic hydrocarbons (PAH) and oxides in urban airborne particulates, *Environ. Int.*, 2, 37, 1979.

77. **Schoeny, R. and Warshawsky, D.,** Mutagenicity of 7H-dibenzo[*c,g*]carbazole and metabolites in *Salmonella typhimurium*, *Mutat. Res.*, 188, 275, 1987.

78. **Parks, W. C., Schurdak, M. E., Randerath, K., Maher, V. M., and McCormick, J. J.,** Human cell-mediated cytotoxicity, mutagenicity, and DNA adduct formation of 7H-dibenzo[*c,g*]carbazole and its *N*-methyl derivative in diploid human fibroblasts, *Cancer Res.*, 46, 4706, 1986.

79. **Perin, F., Valero, D., Thybaud-Lambay, V., Plessis, M. J., and Zajdela, F.,** Organ-specific, carcinogenic dibenzo[c,g]carbazole derivatives: discriminative response in *S. typhimurium* TA100 mutagenesis modulated by subcellular fractions of mouse liver, *Mutat. Res.*, 196, 15, 1988.

80. **Bonin, A. M., Rosario, C. A., Duke, C. C., Baker, R. S. U., Ryan, A. J., and Holder, G. M.,** The mutagenicity of dibenz[a,j] acridine, some metabolites and other derivatives in bacteria and mammalian cells, *Carcinogenesis*, 10, 1079, 1989.

81. **Wogan, G. N.,** Markers of exposure to carcinogens: methods for human biomonitoring, *J. Am. Coll. Toxicol.*, 8, 871, 1989.

82. **van de Poll, M. L. M., van der Hulst, D. A. M., Tates, A. D., Mulder, G. J., and Meerman, J. H. N.,** The role of specific DNA adducts in the induction of mucro-nuclei by *N*-hydroxy-2-acetylaminofluorene in rat liver *in vivo*, *Carcinogenesis*, 10, 717, 1989.

83. **van de Poll, M. L. M., van der Hulst, D. A. M., Tates, A. D., Mulder, G. J., and Meerman, J. H. N.,** Correlation between clastogenicity and promotion activity in liver carcinogenesis by *N*-hydroxy-2-acetyl-aminofluorene, *N*-hydroxy-4′-fluoro-4-acetylaminobiphenyl and *N*-hydroxy-4-acetylaminobiphenyl, *Carcinogenesis*, 11, 333, 1990.

84. **Talaska, G., Au, W. W., Ward, J. B., Jr., Randerath, K., and Legator, M. S.,** The correlation between DNA adducts and chromosomal aberrations in the target organ of benzidine exposed, partially hepatectomized mice, *Carcinogenesis*, 8, 1899, 1987.

85. **Ross, R. K., Yuan, J.-M., Yu, M. C., Wogan, G. N., Qian, G.-S., Tu, J.-T., Groopman, J. D., Gao, Y.-T., and Henderson, B. E.,** Urinary aflatoxin biomarkers and risk of hepatocellular carcinoma, *Lancet*, 339, 943, 1992.

86. **Schurdak, M. E. and Randerath, K.,** Tissue specific DNA adduct formation in mice treated with the environmental carcinogen 7H-dibenzo[c,g]carbazole, *Carcinogenesis*, 6, 1271, 1985.

87. **Roh, J. H., Schamer, M., Reilman, R., Warshawsky, D., and Talaska, G.,** Identification of DNA adduct of 7H-dibenzo [c,g]carbazole and dibenz[a,j]acridine in the mouse following topical application, paper presented at AIH Conference, Boston, MA, May 30 to June 3, 1992.

88. **Li, D., Xu, D., and Randerath, K.,** Species and tissues specificites of I-compounds as contrasted with carcinogen adducts in liver, kidney, and skin DNA of Sprague-Dawley rats, ICR mice and Syrian hamsters, *Carcinogenesis*, 11, 2227, 1990.

89. **Roh, J.-H., Schamer, M., Reilman, R., Xue, W., Warshawsky, D., and Talaska, G.,** ^{32}P-Postlabeling analysis of dibenz[a,j] acridine DNA adducts in mice: preliminary determination of initial genotoxic metabolites and their effect on biomarker levels, *Int. Arch. Occup. Health*, 65, 99, 1993.

90. **Talaska, G., Roh, J., Schamer, M., Reilman, R., Xue, W., and Warshawsky, D.,** ^{32}P-Postlabeling analysis of dibenz[a,j] acridine DNA adducts in mice: identification of proximate metabolites, *Chem. Biol. Interact.*, 95, 161, 1995.

91. **Schurdak, M. E. and Randerath, K.,** Effects of route of administration on tissue distribution of DNA adducts in mice: comparison of 7H-dibenzo[c,g]carbazole, benzo[a]pyrene, and 2-acetylaminofluorene, *Cancer Res.*, 49, 2633, 1989.

92. **Meier, J. and Warshawsky, D.,** Comparison of blood protein and target organ DNA and protein binding following topical application of benzo[a]pyrene and 7H-dibenzo [c,g]carbazole to mice, *Carcinogenesis*, 15, 2233, 1994.

93. **Lindquist, B. E. and Warshawsky, D.,** Binding of 7H-dibenzo[c,g]carbazole to polynucleotides and DNA *in vitro*, *Carcinogenesis*, 10, 2187, 1989.

94. **Schurdak, M. E., Stong, D. B., Warshawsky, D., and Randerath, K.,** ^{32}P-Post-labelling analysis of DNA adduction in mice by synthetic metabolites of the environmetal carcinogen 7H-dibenzo[c,g]carbazole: chromatographic evidence for 3-hydroxy-7H-dibenzo[c,g]carbazole being a proximate

genotoxin in liver but not skin, *Carcinogenesis*, 8, 591, 1987.

95. **Talaska, G., Reilman, R., Schamer, M., Roh, J. H., Xue, W., Fremont, S. L., and Warshawsky, D.,** Tissue distribution of DNA adducts of 7H-dibenzo[*c,g*]carbazole in mice following topical application of the parent compound and its major metabolites, *Chem. Res. Toxicol.*, 7, 374, 1994.

96. **Schurdak, M. E., Stong, D. B., Warshawsky, D., and Randerath, K.,** *N*-methylation reduces the DNA-binding of 7H-dibenzo[*c,g*]carbazole ~300-fold in mouse liver but only ~2-fold in skin: possible correlation with carcinogenic activity, *Carcinogenesis*, 8, 1405, 1987.

97. **Warshawsky, D., Fremont, S., Xue, W., Schneider, J., Jaeger, M., Collins, T., Reilman, R., O'Connor, P., and Talaska, G.,** Target organ specificity for *N*-heterocyclic aromatics, *Polycyclic Aromatic Compd.*, 6, 27, 1994.

98. **Perin-Roussel, O., Perin, F., Barat, N., Plessis, M. J., and Zajdela, F.,** Interaction of 7H-dibenzo[*c,g*]carbazole and its organ specific derivatives with hepatic mitochondrial and nuclear DNA in the mouse, *Environ. Mol. Mutagen.*, 25, 202, 1995.

99. **Warshawsky, D., Livingston, G. K., Fonouni-Fard, M., and LaDow, K.,** Induction of micronuclei and sister chromatid exchanges by polycyclic and *N*-heterocyclic aromatic hydrocarbons in cultured human lymphocytes, *Environ. Mol. Mutagen.*, 26, 109, 1995.

100. **Krishnan, S. P. and Warshawsky, D.,** Relationship between formation of carcinogen-DNA adducts and micronuclei in mouse keratinocytes exposed to carcinogens, paper presented at meeting of Society of Toxicology, Baltimore, MD, March 5 to 9, 1995.

101. **O'Connor, P., Warshawsky, D., and Talaska, G.,** Chromatographic comparison of polynucleotide adducts resulting from *in vitro* and *in vivo* activation of 7H-dibenzo[*c,g*]carbazole, paper presented at Society of Toxicology Annual Meeting, Dallas, March 13 to 17, 1994.

CONCLUDING REMARKS

The past 4 years have brought major advances in the analytical chemistry of tobacco-specific N-nitrosamines (TSNA). Brunnemann et al. reported that the bioavailability of tobacco-specific N-nitrosamines (TSNA), especially that of 4-(methylnitrosamino)-1-(3-pyridyl)-1-butanone (NNK), is greater than has been previously estimated on the basis of conventional organic solvent extraction methods. Incubation of saliva with snuff and subsequent extraction with organic solvents does not lead to a point at which TSNA extraction ceases; however, supercritical fluid extraction (SFE) with carbon dioxide containing 10% methanol results in the complete removal of all TSNA. Research by Idris with scientists at the International Cancer Center in Lyon as well as with scientists at the American Health Foundation has shown that *toombak,* a home-made snuff used in northern Sudan, contains at least 100-fold higher concentrations of carcinogenic TSNA than the commercial snuff brands in the U.S. and Sweden. The high exposure of the *toombak* chewers is also reflected in the levels of TSNA found in their saliva. In addition, biomarker studies have shown that *toombak* chewers have very high levels of hemoglobin adducts of N'-nitrosonornicotine (NNN) and NNK and of the urinary metabolites of NNK. The TSNA analysis of indoor air can serve as a marker for the degree of pollution by tobacco-specific carcinogens. Although gas chromatography-thermal energy analyzer (GC-TEA) can presently detect down to 0.5 ng of TSNA per injection, this detection limit is not sensitive enough to quantify individual TSNA in small samples of physiological fluids, such as bronchial lavage or cervical mucus. More sensitive methods are now needed for the quantitative analyses of TSNA as well as for the determination of their metabolites.

Amin et al. described the various methods employed for the syntheses of TSNA and their metabolites and adducts. Providing such compounds fills a great need for research in biochemistry and molecular biology. Efforts are now underway to synthesize TSNA adducts with DNA. The highly advanced organic synthetic methods enable the preparation of various N-nitrosamines that are structurally related to TSNA. Amin et al. discussed this aspect by way of syntheses of the analogs of NNN. The newly synthesized NNN-related nitrosamines will lead to bioassays and to the elucidation of those structural features that influence the carcinogenic potential of TSNA.

The study group of Nair et al. with Bartsch as senior scientist presents an overview of our present knowledge on the endogenous formation of carcinogenic N-nitrosamines, especially as it relates to TSNA in tobacco smokers, snuff dippers, and chewers of tobacco and of betel quid mixtures with tobacco. Whereas it has been clearly demonstrated that TSNA are formed during the chewing of tobacco, the question about endogenous formation of NNK from nicotine in smokers is still not fully elucidated. Tobacco contains the noncarcinogenic N-nitrosamino acid 4-(methylnitrosamino)-4-(3-pyridyl) butyric acid (*iso*-NNAC), which is formed during tobacco processing. Because *iso*-NNAC is not formed during smoking and only minute amounts of it are transferred from tobacco into cigarette smoke (<1.0%), it has been suggested that the urinary concentration of *iso*-NNAC could serve as an indicator of the endogenous formation of TSNA from nicotine. Nair et al. reviewed the literature on this subject and concluded that *iso*-NNAC is most likely formed endogenously from nicotine; however, further studies are needed to confirm this. An important aspect of the endogenous formation of nitrosamines, including TSNA, concerns the conditions during inflammatory processes. NO' is known to be endogenously generated during inflammation, during infections by bacteria, parasites, or viruses. However, so far, model studies have been carried out with rodents that are able to synthesize ascorbic acid, an inhibitor of endogenous NO' formation during infection. Obviously, the human setting must be more closely mimicked with studies in animal models that are not confounded by ascorbic acid generation.

Hecht discussed the metabolism of the highly carcinogenic NNK in laboratory animals and humans as well as the involvement of enzymes in the bioactivation of this TSNA. Of special interest is the observation that the detoxification of NNK occurs via its reduction product 4-(methylnitrosamino)-1-(3-pyridyl)-1-butanol (NNAL), which is excreted in the urine as a glucuronide (NNAL-Gluc) and as a free secondary alcohol, NNAL. Like NNK, NNAL is a lung carcinogen. The urinary excretion ratio of NNAL-Gluc to NNAL may indicate the lung cancer risk of a smoker. Biomarker studies with different populations of smokers are now underway to enable an evaluation of this concept. Recently, the α-glucuronide of the α-hydroxylation product of NNK, 4-(hydroxymethylnitrosamino)-1-(3-pyridyl)-1-butanone, has been detected *in vitro* with hepatocytes and also *in vivo* in the urine of rats. This finding shows that this glucuronide of hydroxymethyl NNK presents a stable form of the activated NNK that may be involved in NNK carcinogenicity. Hecht also discussed the present state of knowledge of the DNA and protein adduct formation with NNK metabolites in rodents and in humans. Current data strongly suggest that the methylation of DNA as well as pyridyloxobutylation play important roles in the carcinogenicity of NNK. The methylation product O^6-mG-DNA induces K-ras oncogene activation in codon 12 with GGT-GAT mutations in the lungs of mice and hamsters. In smokers with lung adenocarcinoma, 24% have been found to have mutations in codon 12. Of these, 19% had GGT-GAT transitions and 16% showed GGT-GTT transversions. In the mouse, the NNK pyridyloxobutylation of DNA leads to both G to A transitions and G to T transversions in codon 12 of the K-ras oncogene. Studies of the effects of NNK on mutations of the p53 tumor suppressor gene in lung tumors are underway.

Gupta et al. presented an overview on the occurrence of oral cancer as it relates to tobacco use. In the U.S., about 90% of deaths from lung cancer among men and 79% of those among women are associated with smoking. In India, 10% of about 665,000 new cases of cancer are neoplasms in the oral cavity. Extensive epidemiological studies have shown that the chewing of betel quid with tobacco is a major etiological factor for oral cancer in India in other countries in Southeast Asia. The authors reviewed the scientific literature and concluded that the carcinogenic TSNA are a major etiological factor in cancer of the oral cavity among chewers of betel quid with tobacco.

During the last 2 to 3 decades, the mortality from adenocarcinoma of the peripheral lung among smokers in the U.S. has increased significantly more than that from squamous cell carcinoma of the lung, especially in male smokers. Hoffmann et al. discussed a hypothesis that may explain this observation. Under standard laboratory smoking conditions, the sales-weighted average "tar" and nicotine yields of U.S. cigarettes have decreased since 1955 from 38 and 2.7 mg to 13.5 and 0.9 mg, respectively. The major factors for these decreases in "tar" and nicotine are the marked increase of the sales of filter cigarettes from 0.5 to more than 97% of all cigarettes currently sold, the use of perforated filter tips, reconstituted tobacco sheets, and expanded tobacco in the cigarette tobacco blend, as well as the increase of the nitrate content in tobacco from about 0.3 to 0.5% to 1.2 to 1.5%. These product changes have caused smokers to draw puffs more intensely and inhale smoke more deeply to reach a physiologically conditioned level of nicotine. The increase of the nitrate content of the tobacco blend reduces the yields of the carcinogenic aromatic hydrocarbons in the smoke significantly; however, it enhances TSNA formation. In a leading U.S. cigarette, the levels of benzo(*a*)pyrene decreased since 1965 from 50 to 20 ng per cigarette, whereas the NNK yields increased from about 110 to 160 ng per cigarette. Thus, when smoking low-yield cigarettes, smokers not only puff more frequently and inhale the smoke more deeply into their lungs, but their peripheral lungs are also exposed to relatively higher doses of the adenocarcinoma-inducing NNK. This concept is currently being explored by assessing puff volume, puff frequency, puff duration, and butt length of individual smokers of cigarettes with low, medium, and high nicotine yields. These assessments are made with a newly developed special device. The parameters determined with this device can be programed into machine-smoking settings, and the chemical analyses of smoke so generated will then reflect more accurately the composition of smoke and dose of carcinogens to which each individual cigarette smoker is exposed. The urine analyses for nicotine, cotinine, NNAL-Gluc, and NNAL will provide additional leads toward interpreting individual rates of metabolism.

Evidently, the symposium presentations point to the need for future studies in tobacco carcinogenesis that focus on the contribution of the TSNA to the carcinogenic potential of smokeless tobacco and tobacco smoke, with studies on biochemical and biological markers.

ACKNOWLEDGMENTS

We express our sincere thanks to the organizers of the 16th International Cancer Congress in New Delhi, India, in October/November 1994, especially to Dr. M. G. Deo, the chairman of the Scientific Program, for allotting time and space for the Symposium on Tobacco-Specific *N*-Nitrosamines. We greatly appreciate the editorial assistance of Ilse Hoffmann and Jennifer Johnting of the American Health Foundation.

Dietrich Hoffman
American Health Foundation
Valhalla, NY

Printed and bound by CPI Group (UK) Ltd, Croydon, CR0 4YY

25/10/2024

01779218-0001